NURTURE

Architecture of Sustainable Design:
The School of Nursing + Student Community Center

ORO *editions*

BNIM Architects
Lake | Flato Architects

NURTURE

Architecture of Sustainable Design:
The School of Nursing + Student Community Center at
The University of Texas Health Science Center at Houston

Steve McDowell + David Lake
Introduction by **Andrew Payne + Rodolphe el-Khoury**

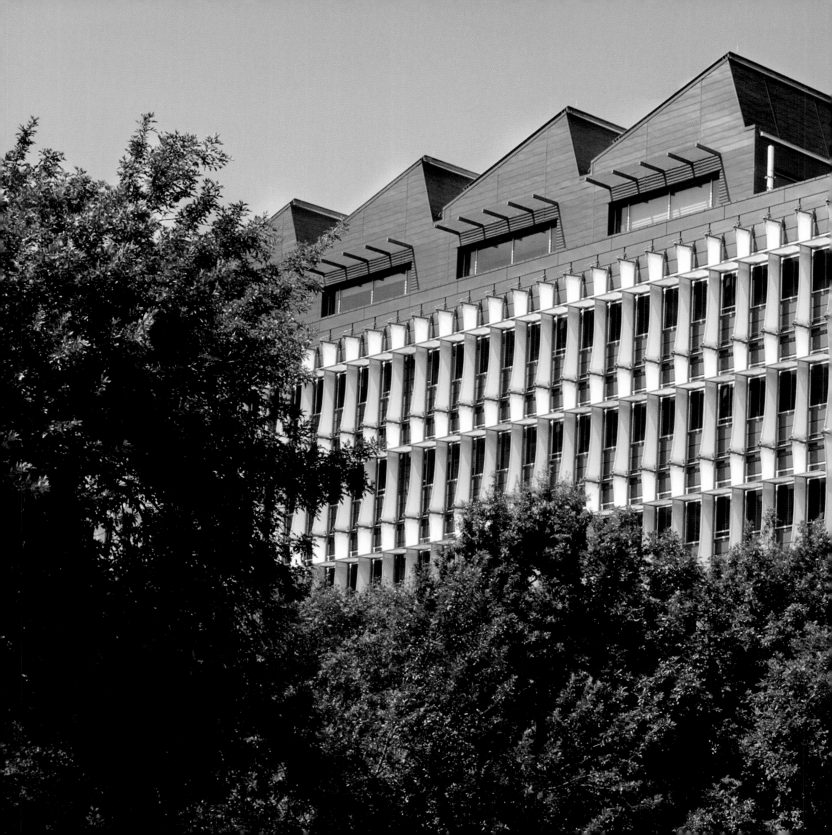

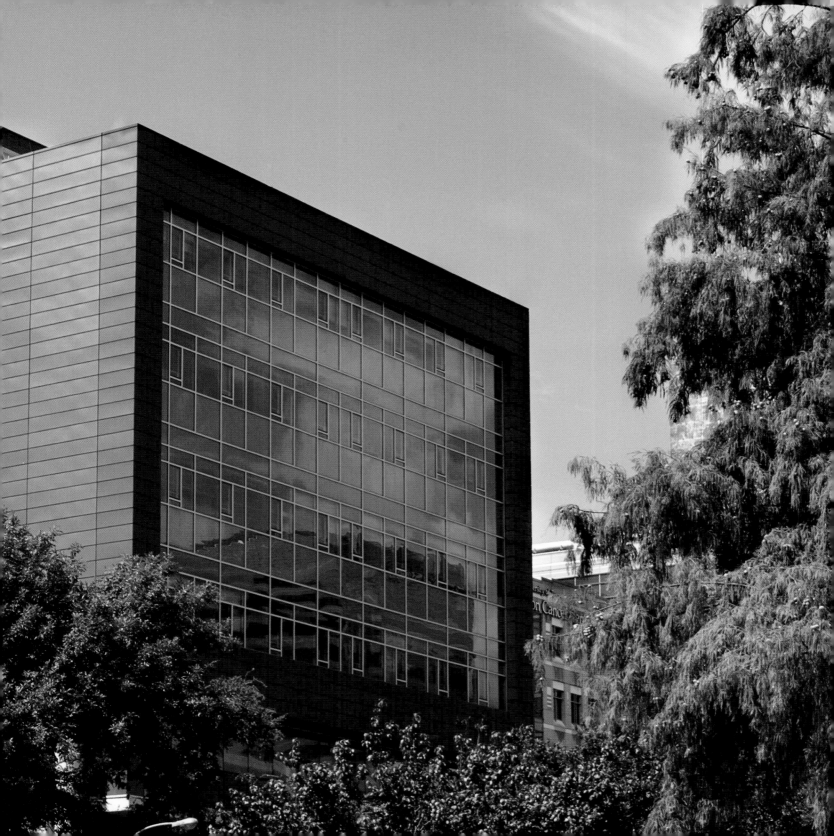

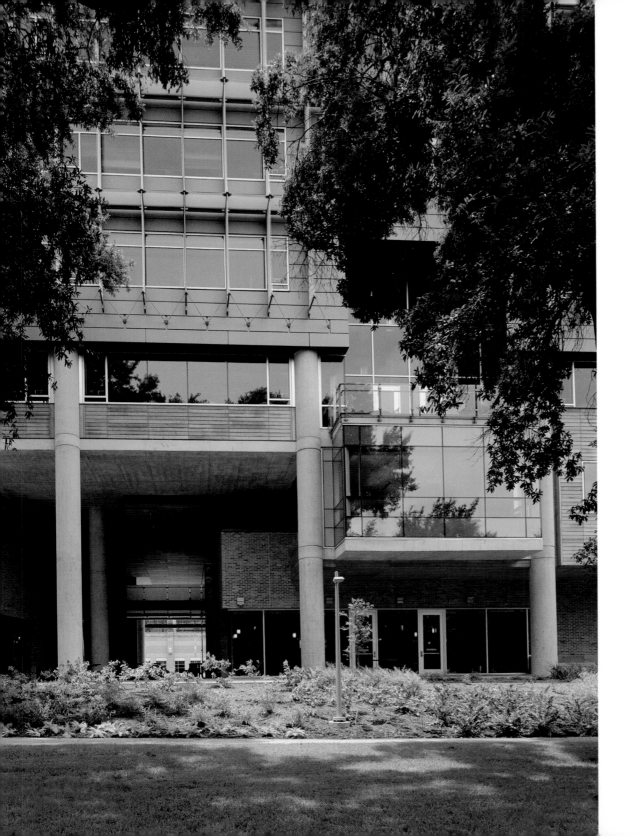

DEDICATION

He who has health has hope, and he who has hope has everything.
—Arabian proverb

This book recognizes the visionary leadership at The University of Texas Health Science Center at Houston, whose marked dedication to creating a benchmark building for pedagogy, sustainability and the pursuit of human health was the central design inspiration.

It has taken numerous individuals with countless innovative ideas and cutting-edge technology to accomplish the project's goals and aspirations. These goals indicate the commendable foresight, the the commitment to excellence and the profound potential that this project has for the future of education, the field of design and the School of Nursing.

When the submission process began in July of 2000, the team commented that this building represented a "turning point." Indeed, as the School of Nursing and Student Community Center opened its doors to students and educators, it was apparent that this turning point was upon us. The influence of this work is certain to ripple outward and impart to others the lessons that have been learned and the examples that have been set for nursing and for sustainable design.

Above all, as a team we are grateful to The University of Texas System and the UT School of Nursing at Houston for allowing us to share in this process of collaboration and discovery. It has been an immensely challenging and deeply rewarding journey—one that we hope will inspire others in their path toward a nurturing architecture.

TABLE OF CONTENTS

	Introduction	12
001	Idea	15
002	Approach + Process	26
003	Place	33
004	Program	39
005	Design Concept	50
006	Envelope Design Concept	59
007	Daylighting Design	74
008	Sustainable Design Strategies	85
1	Sustainable Sites	86
2	Water Efficiency	91
3	Indoor Environmental Quality	94
4	Energy + Atmosphere	99
5	Materials + Resources	102
6	Innovation + Design Process	106
009	Design	111

Generous Pragmatism in BNIM Architects + Lake|Flato's School of Nursing

Introduction by Andrew Payne + Rodolphe el-Khoury

Behind the recent brouhaha concerning the building as spectacle, the Bilbao effect, as it has come to be known, we can observe the emergence of a new pragmatism in contemporary architecture, a concern with how well buildings perform in response to the full range of social and ecological processes they are called on to organize. The work of BNIM Architects and Lake|Flato makes them implicit advocates of this pragmatism in which what a building can do matters as much as what it looks like. Their buildings are perhaps best described as instruments or devices whose function is to instill in their occupants an ethos of engaged propinquity in settings that bring the convenience and intensity of the artificial environment into intimate proximity with the amenities associated with the natural surrounding. What is more, their buildings perform this complex function in accordance with practices designed not only to minimize negative ecological consequences of construction, but also to ensure each building's ongoing contribution to the ecosystem in which it performs. In view of this ecological emphasis, we can be more precise about the building's instrumentality: they are biotechnical instruments, living machines. Having said that, what makes these buildings especially compelling is the way in which this ecologically spirited instrumentality, fashioned over fifty years of collective practice, is inflected by a generosity toward the lived character of organized human affairs. In these buildings, the minutiae of everyday life are treated not as obstacles to architectural invention; they are, rather, invention's justifying occasion. Far from being overlooked, the normative routines of contemporary professional existence are consistently embraced by BNIM and Lake|Flato as so many opportunities for bringing the built environment into a deeper attunement with our collective desire for convenience and delight.

Such commitments and inclinations enabled the successful collaboration with Lake|Flato, with whom they joined forces in designing the School of Nursing and Student Community Center at The University of Texas Health Science Center at Houston.

Here, the synergy between like-minded firms produces one of the finest demonstrations of generous pragmatism: technical efficacy in optimizing performance coupled with an aesthetic commitment to sustaining everyday pleasures.

The aesthetic of the technical instrument is an aesthetic of self-effacement, and this building as biotechnical instrument is no exception to that rule. On first glance, it is a box set squarely on its site, a box among the many boxes that comprise the Houston landscape. This continuity with the idiom of its place is in fact a form of camouflage, however, for unlike the boxes that surround it, which are pretty dumb, this box is a clever box— clever enough to nest within its restrained massing a series of ingenuously simple devices for bringing organization, space and light to the event of human congregation. Approaching the building on axis, one sees this aesthetic of self-effacement literalized in the void that penetrates the building's cube at its center. The insertion of this void has at least two effects. First, it nests an exterior space at the heart of the building's interior, emblematizing the building's larger strategy of engagement with its surroundings. Second, it transforms the building into a monumental frame or proscenium that serves to put the visitor, arriving from a landscape composed of parking lots and dumb-box building stock, in immediate contact with what is unquestionably the site's chief aesthetic amenity, the park lying on its north side. The "breezeway" that this piercing of the center of the building's interior volume provides also serves as a shaded space for public congregation, an alternative to the sun-exposed space of the park onto which it gives way. Hence, the breezeway serves as a device for putting otherwise disjointed things in a relationship of vital proximity to one another: events of arrival and events of occupation; artificial and living systems; interior and exterior spaces; openness and purposiveness; optical drift and spatial definition. In that sense, also, this device is emblematic of the architects' larger commitments, for in their version of the building as living machine, the mechanic operation always involves bringing two or more persons or things into a relationship of adaptive advantage. This relational strategy concerns more than merely placing the site's amenities at the immediate disposal of those occupying the building's interior—it also involves enlisting the building in a re-orchestration of the elements composing the urban context, establishing new relationships and hierarchical dynamics between those elements. In the hermetic and atomized landscape of Houston, where the operative logic linking persons and things remains largely hidden from view, the breezeway acts as a kind of urban ventilation system: a system for circulating light, air and space, to be sure, but also for circulating common sense, a degree of collective intelligence concerning our relationship to our immediate surroundings.

The instrumental approach to built form is also apparent in the treatment of the School of Nursing's façades. That approach eschews any attempt to convey an integral gestalt, in favor of a faceted approach in which each elevation responds to the conditions peculiar to its orientation. Whereas the front elevation opens the building to the park as the site's chief amenity, the other elevations are designed to maximize and manage sunlight while limiting passive heat gain during the hot summer days. This strategy of employing the façade as a filter for letting in light and keeping out heat is repeated on the building's roof. Replete with a network of skylights and reflectors working to coordinate natural light and shade in the building below, this roof truly does manifest the oft invoked but seldom realized ideal of a fifth façade. On all elevations, the cubic massing of the building is echoed in a strategy of varied reticulation that, in keeping with the instrumental aesthetic described above, prizes the flexibility of operative configurations over more classical compositional strategies.

The advantages of this pragmatic strategy are immediately and powerfully felt on the building's interior. True to the aesthetic of self-effacement, BNIM and Lake|Flato have taken pains to design not merely the built object, but the atmosphere it contains.

Using advanced digital simulation technologies, the architects have calculated the quality of light and its associated ambiance with a precision generally reserved for more tangible media like glass, steel and stone. As a result, the most memorable feature of the building may be the most immaterial. Long after visitors have forgotten the self-effacing elegance of the object, they are likely to retain a strong impression of the atmosphere of airy transparence this object evinces and contains.

This emphasis on delivering natural light, so very apparent in the treatment of elevations, is echoed in the sectional strategy, which is organized around the provision of atria that extend deep into the heart of the building along both horizontal and vertical axes. It is in section that the box most fully reveals itself as a permeable framework penetrated by shafts of light. These strategies lend to the building a sense of openness and transparency that is simultaneously pastoral and urbane. This is a generous conception of the contemporary institutional building, one in which the vicarious social pleasures lining the daily performance of our professional routines are not cynically theatricalized—as in so much contemporary architecture—but rather, recast in the light of an entirely pragmatic and contemporary Arcadian ideal.

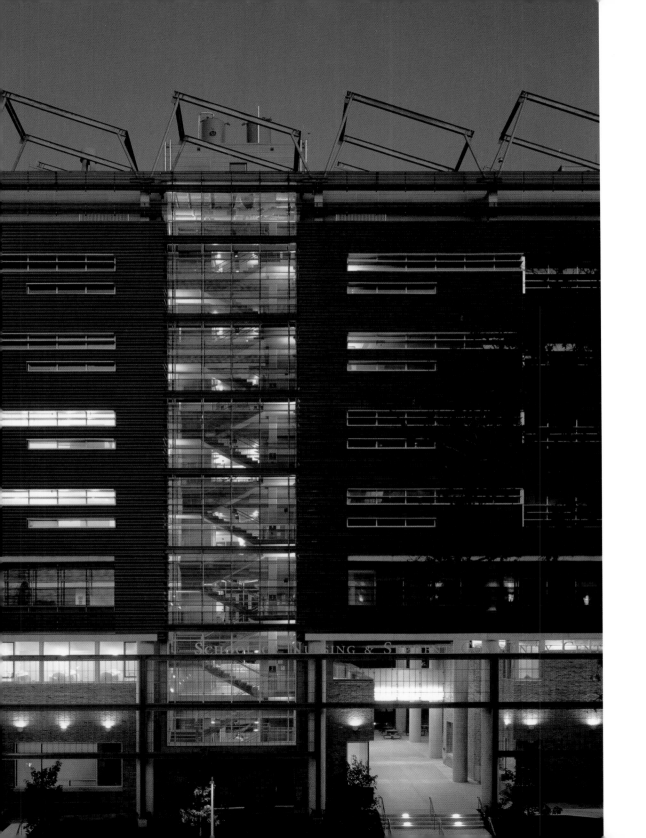

001 IDEA

"Nursing is not only scientific and knowledge-based; there is also caring and compassion—the healing component. So we wanted a building that feels like a nurturing environment the minute you enter it."

Patricia L. Starck, D.S.N.
Dean, The UT School of Nursing at Houston

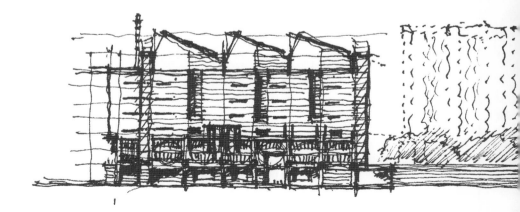

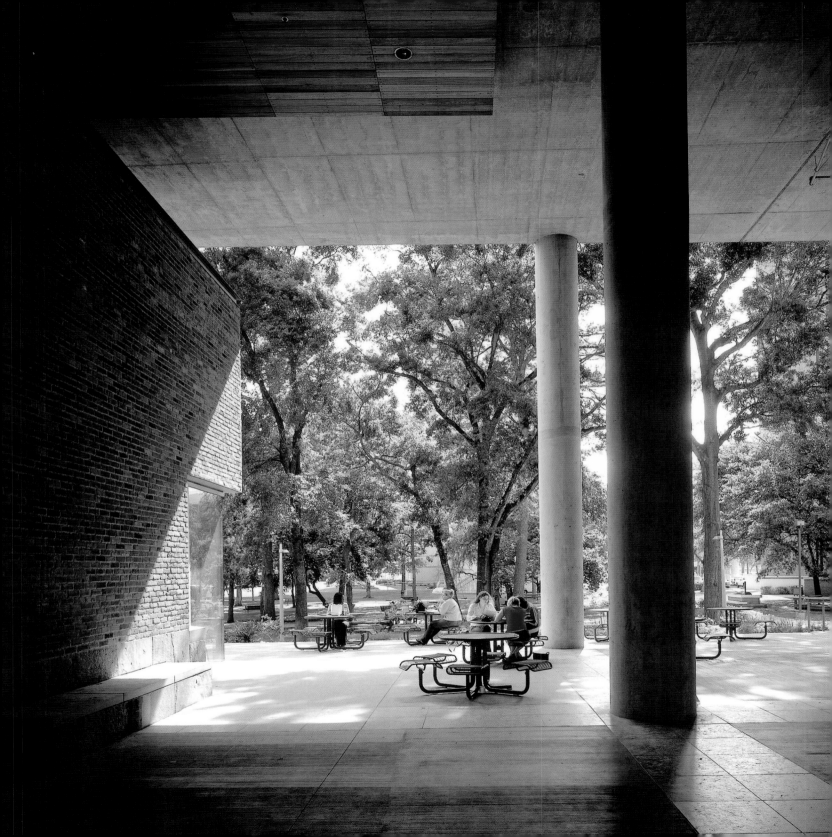

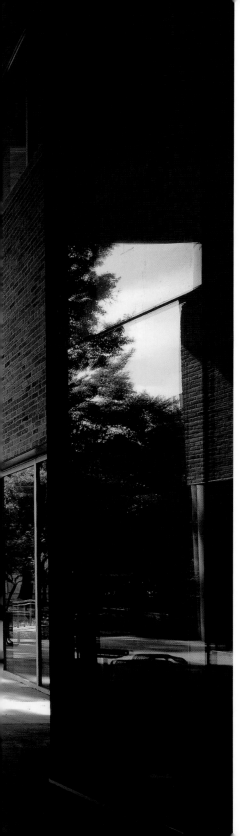

The School of Nursing and Student Community Center had an important role in providing a portal to The University of Texas Health Science Center campus and a connection to the Texas Medical Center. The university lacked a cohesive campus and, therefore, the new building would be a welcoming presence and serve as a home for the wider university community. The ensuing building was designed to integrate seamlessly with its site and impart a sense of place that would become a heart for the campus. The building would function as a community center uniting academic and social interactions, while the adjacent park would serve as a quad in this nontraditional campus setting. State-of-the-art classrooms, laboratories, study carrels, an auditorium, café, bookstore and other spaces were established to serve the educational and community needs of the larger population. To balance the needs of students, faculty and the community, it was decided that the building and its landscape should be a warm, inviting and state-of-the-art environment for learning, research and student service. It should be a model for the integration of building purpose, program and academics.

Conservation of all types of resources is an important mandate of the university. The building owners understood that meeting their fiduciary responsibilities did not end with the building's design and construction costs, which represent less than 20% of the total cost of ownership. This building was challenged to do more. It was to set new standards for energy and be extremely responsible in its water-management practices. Savings realized from the building's reduced operating costs would make it possible to redirect dollars to the core mission of the university.

The team hoped that this building would become a model facility, a paradigm with enough presence and vigor that it would influence the design and construction of university architecture and, perhaps, impact future buildings with its valuable examples. The ensuing building is designed as a pedagogical model of wellness, comfort, flexibility, environmental stewardship and fiscal responsibility.

PREVIOUS
West elevation and breezeway
with central stair designed to encourage
visibility of surrounding context.

LEFT
Breezeway view into Grant Fay Park,
the heart of the UTHSC-H campus.

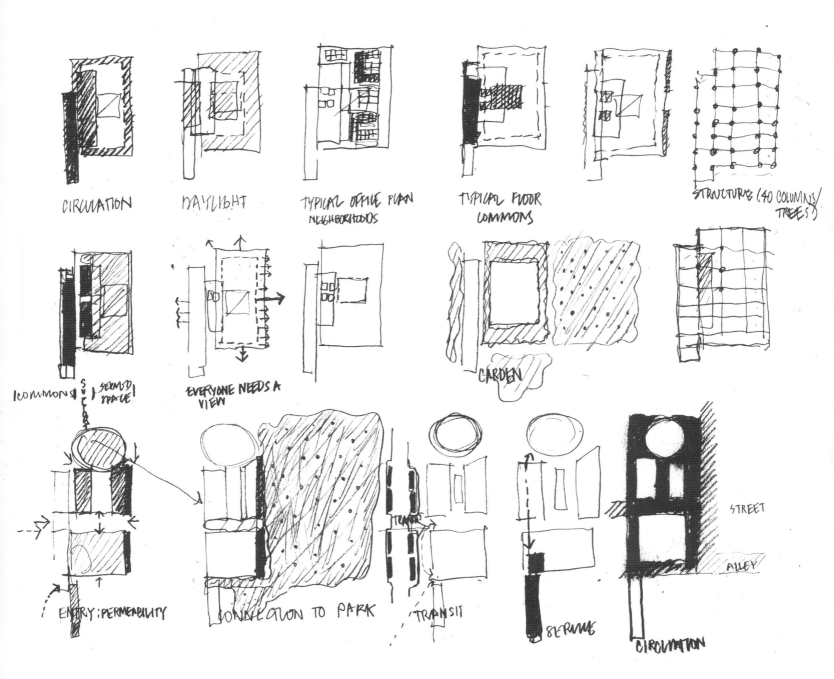

CIRCULATION

DAYLIGHT

TYPICAL OFFICE PLAN
NEIGHBORHOODS

TYPICAL FLOOR
COMMONS

STRUCTURE (40 COLUMNS/
TREES?)

COMMONS | SECOND SPACE

EVERYONE NEEDS A VIEW

GARDEN

ENTRY : PERMEABILITY

CONNECTION TO PARK

TRANSIT

SERVING

STREET

ALLEY

CIRCULATION

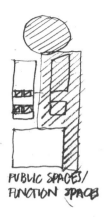

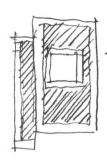

PUBLIC SPACES/
FUNCTION SPACE

COMFORT ZONE

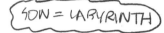

SOW = LABYRINTH

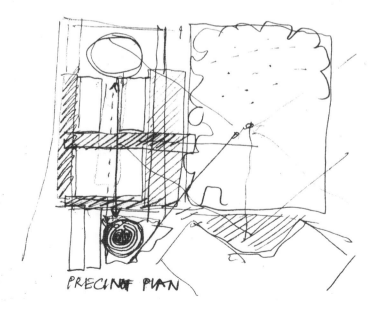

PRECINCT PLAN

LEFT
Integrating program and systems
with the site to create a learning
environment that features:

· Daylighting
· Flexibility
· Community
· Connections
· Function
· Connection to park
· Permeability
· Symbol
· Pedagogy

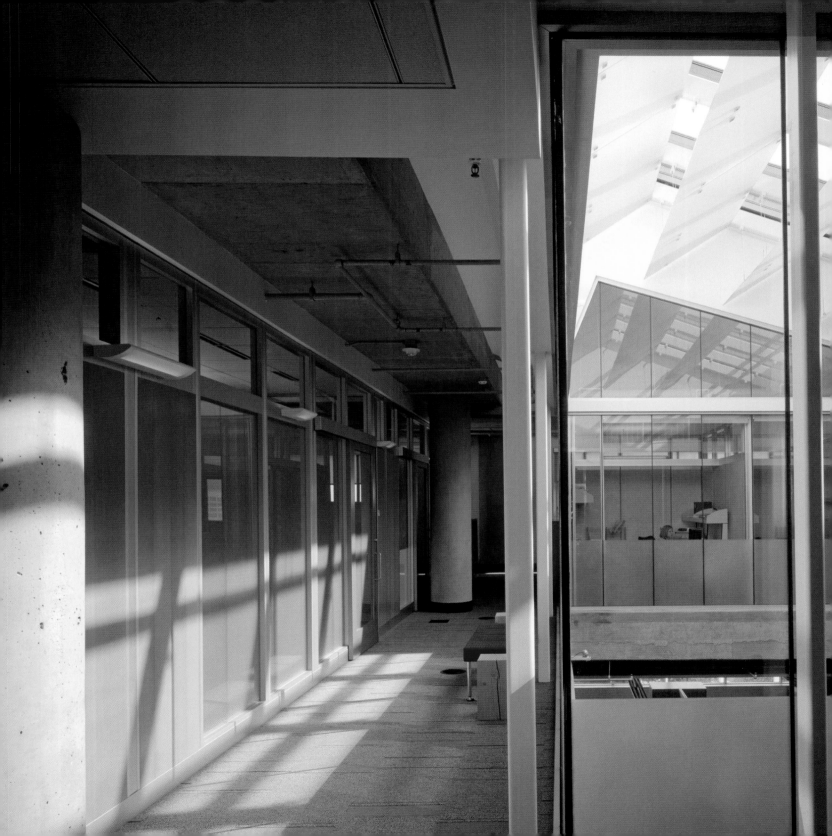

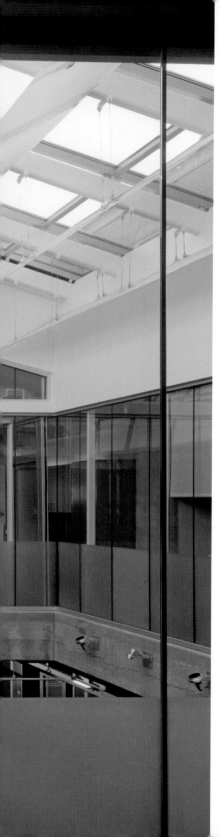

LEFT
Workplace atria showing surrounding
private offices, demountable partitions
and clerestory glazing. The workplace
maximizes both daylighting and flexibility.

The School of Nursing + Student Community Center
was designed and constructed:

- To endure for more than 100 years as a flexible and
  adaptable facility that evolves with the changing needs
  of the school.

- To uplift the spirit of the dwellers with interior spaces
  that harvest daylighting, reflect timeless design and are
  welcoming and comfortable.

- To respect its surroundings and thus create an academic
  climate that inspires creativity, collaboration, collegiality
  and learning.

- To minimize the negative effect of the structure on its
  natural site.

- To contain the best workmanship by partnering with
  companies that use only proven, state-of-the-art equipment
  and materials.

- To sustain economic efficiencies by mandating that utility
  costs should be 70% less than the adjacent University of
  Texas School of Public Health constructed in 1977 and
  construction costs not to exceed 105% of the cost of a
  conventionally constructed building.

- To incorporate all natural opportunities presented by
  the physical site and to design economy into long-term
  maintenance and operational costs.

- To extol the indigenous environment by landscaping exterior
  spaces with plants and trees that are natural to the
  Houston area and require minimal care, chemicals and water.

- To utilize non-toxic materials and take advantage of
  renewable energy sources.

- To apply life-cycle costing in evaluating design strategies.

- To use natural, recycled and reclaimed materials
  from sources and manufacturers in Texas to the fullest
  extent possible.

- To incorporate systems into the infrastructure that ensure
  efficient use of resources and drive recycling.

LEFT
An early concept sketch defines the
primary design strategies.

RIGHT
The building's rainscreen skin appears delicate
in contrast with the solid podium; however its
durable nature serves multiple functions in the
Houston climate including insulation, shading
and resistance to moisture.

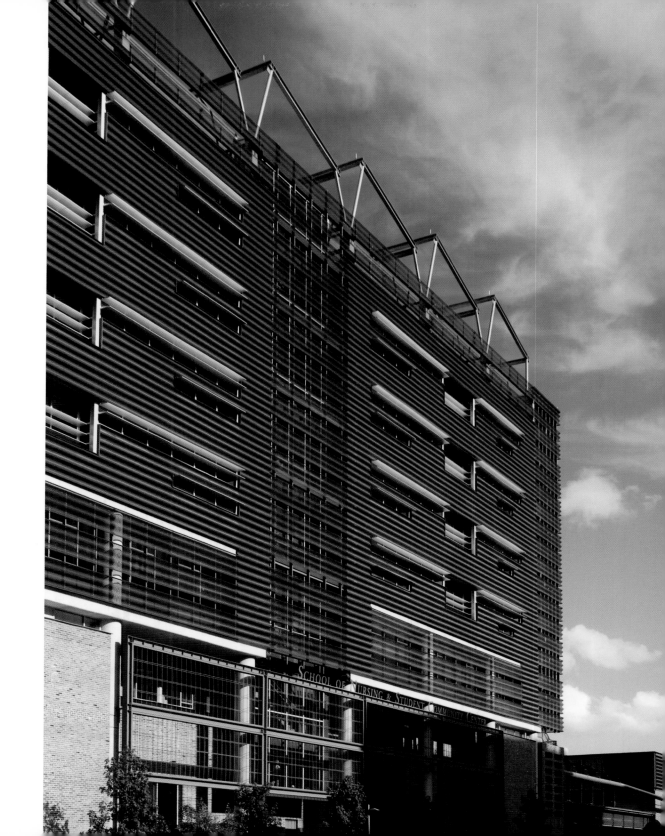

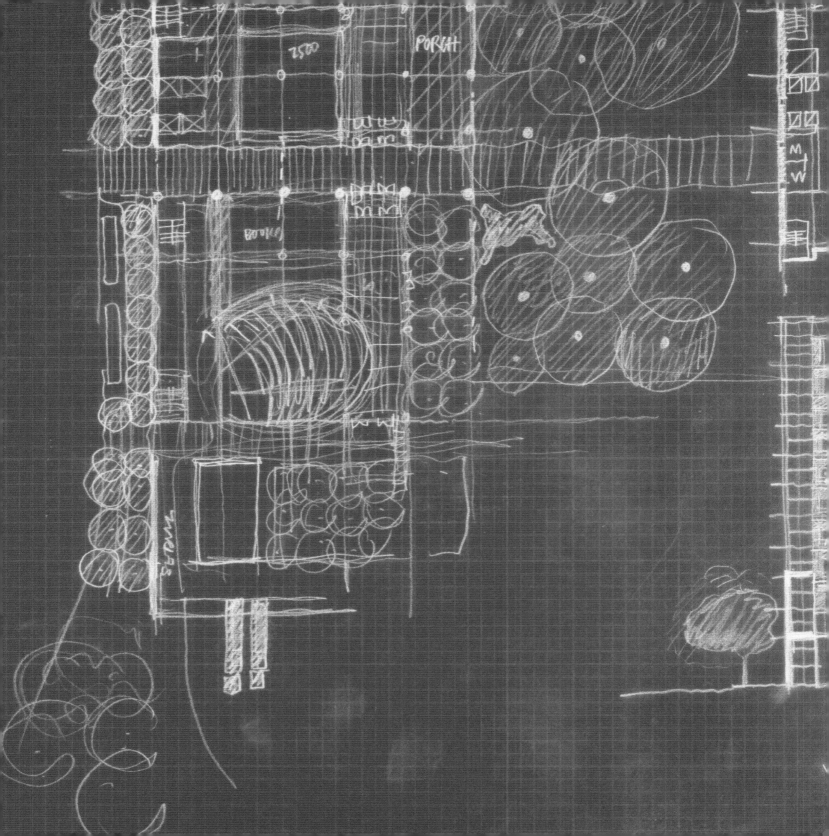

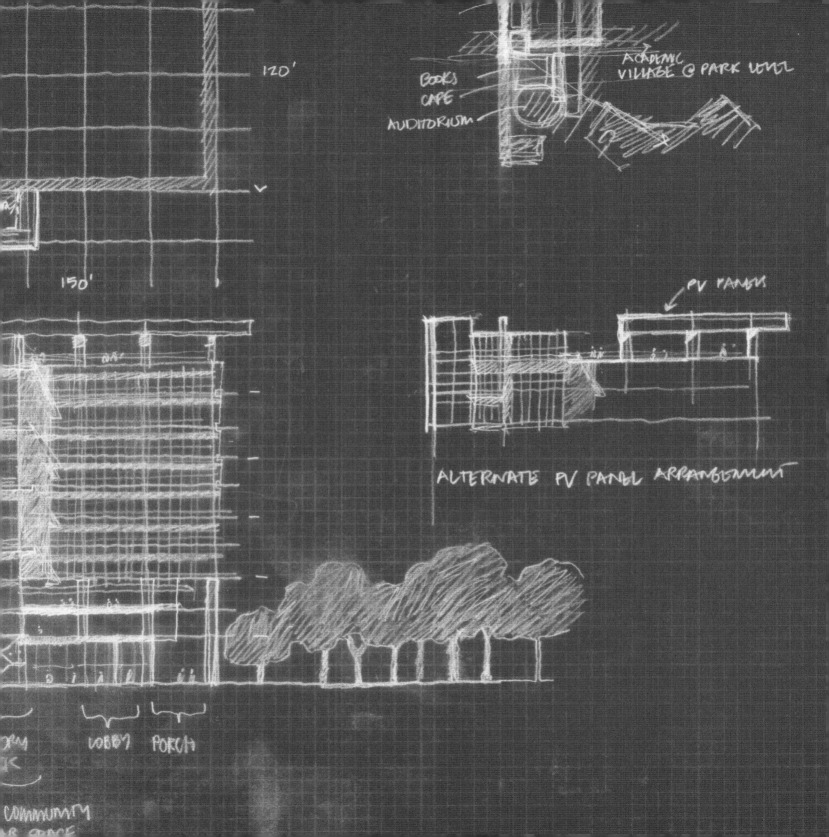

120'

150'

BOOKS
CAFE
AUDITORIUM

ACADEMIC
VILLAGE @ PARK LEVEL

PV PANELS

ALTERNATE PV PANEL ARRANGEMENT

LOBBY   PORCH

COMMUNITY

OO2 APPROACH + PROCESS :
INTEGRATED DESIGN

To fully comprehend what was possible, an unusually high level of participation from the client and users was required. Representatives from seventeen firms and an equally large client group worked together to set and refine goals and test strategies from the very beginning. The entire team worked together in a highly collaborative manner to achieve the goals for the project. An open, inclusive and integrated process transformed the design from simply an idea into the exemplary building that stands today.

The integrated design process is founded on a method of holistic thinking achieved through both organized collaboration between disciplines and through the interweaving and *interconnectivity* of building systems.

The initial project meeting gathered over fifty attendees, each of whom was necessary to ensure that each aspect of the program was considered and specific responses to that program were devised.

In the initial design charrette, the design team collectively agreed to emphasize performance and function first and foremost. The team focused on fresh approaches that saved energy, provided more comfort and control for the users, simplified building operations and made for a more adaptable and lasting building. To confirm these decisions, life-cycle costing was applied, and the results of the studies supported the long-term advantages of an asymmetric envelope design and numerous other sustainable design strategies. In addition to setting critical milestones, concepts were rigorously tested at every level. Each major building system was analyzed, and potential solutions were brainstormed by users, facilities staff, construction managers, engineers and architects. This method continued through the evolution of the design phases, ultimately achieving a healthy, productive and nurturing building.

RIGHT
Three identical daylit atria link the top three office and administrative floors, bringing daylight to the core.

OVERLEAF
Design development charrette.

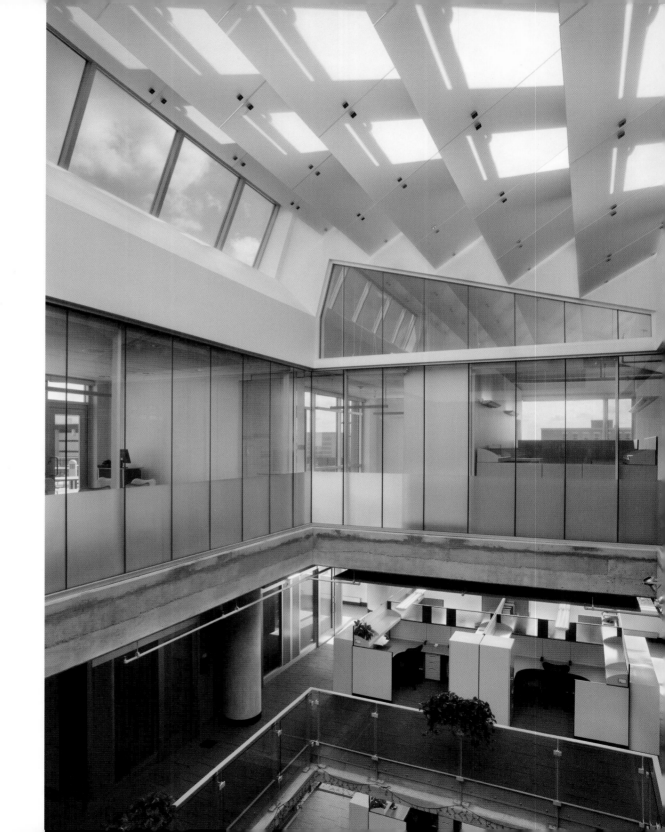

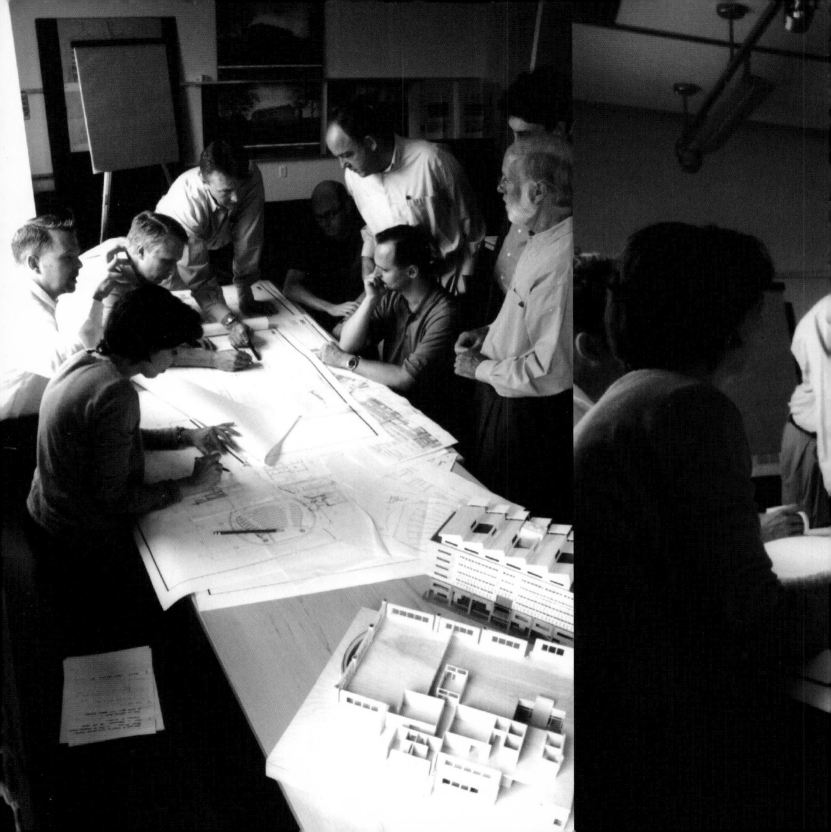

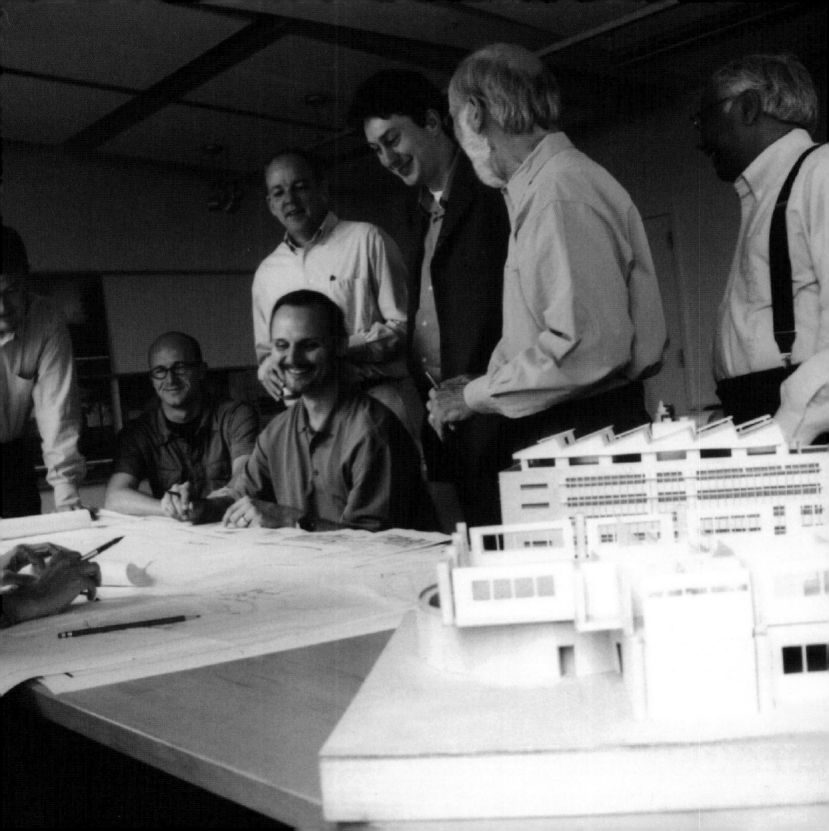

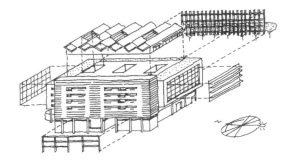

FIVE FAÇADES

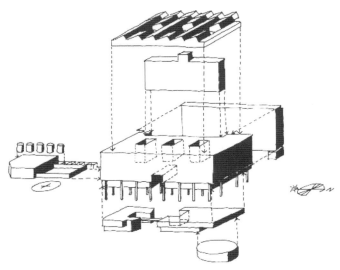

ARCHITECTURAL COMPONENTS

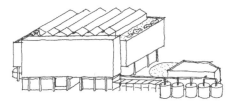

RAINWATER COLLECTION

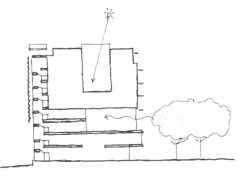

DAYLIGHT PENETRATION

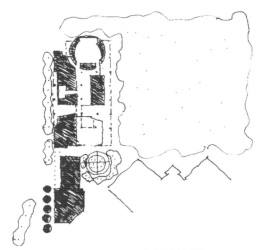

GROUND-FLOOR PUBLIC SPACE

ABOVE
Architectural diagrams showing the integration
of building systems integrated into the façade.

RIGHT
Aerial photo of nursing school shows adjacency
to Grant Fay Park, showing six shed roofs and
three atria. The roofs were designed to support
a future photovoltaic array.

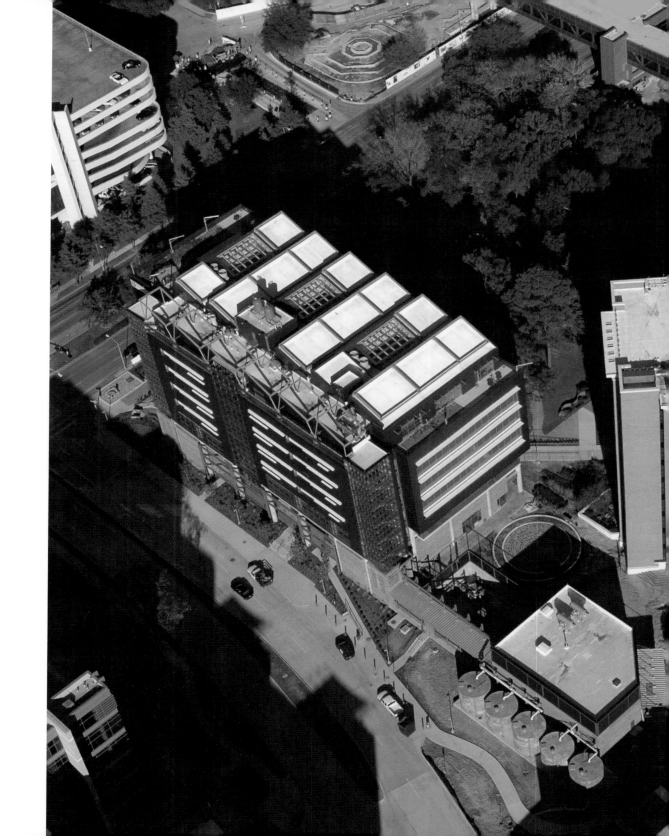

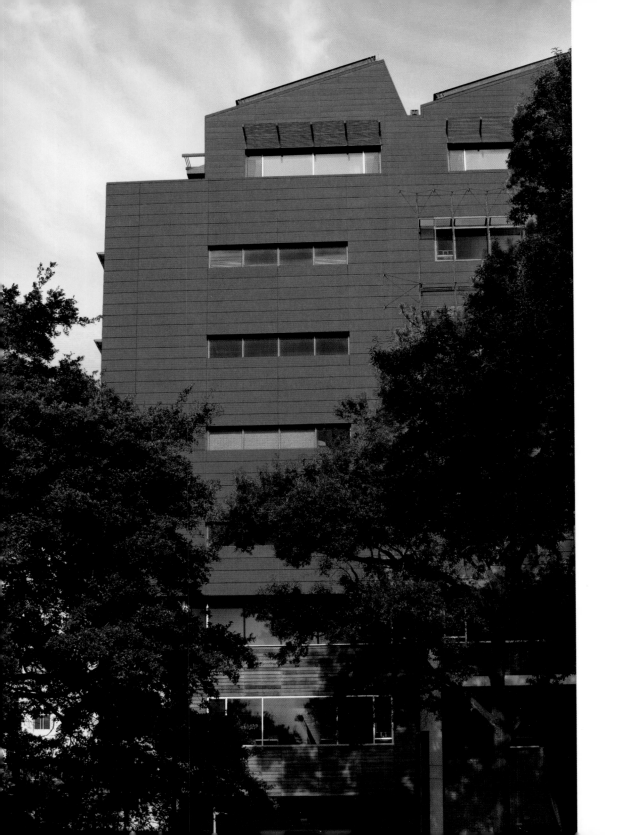

003 PLACE

HOUSTON

Houston is located in a difficult climate where hot, humid summers and mild, temperate winters challenge the built environment with respect to human comfort issues, air quality, periodic flooding and energy conservation.

These conditions place *enormous* demands on buildings and supporting systems, such as mechanical and envelope design.

The climate also challenges the typical sustainable design strategies employed for buildings of this type: fresh air ventilation is difficult to accomplish because of the heat, humidity and poor air quality; the sun can be extreme and difficult to harness for effective interior daylighting; large amounts of rain arrive during relatively short periods of the year, making surplus water available, but requiring greater capacity to store water for use in the dry, hot season; and the area is prone to hurricane conditions that place stress on building and site systems. These issues challenged the design team, but also made it clear why sustainable design strategies were important, not only for this building, but for the environment of the city and beyond.

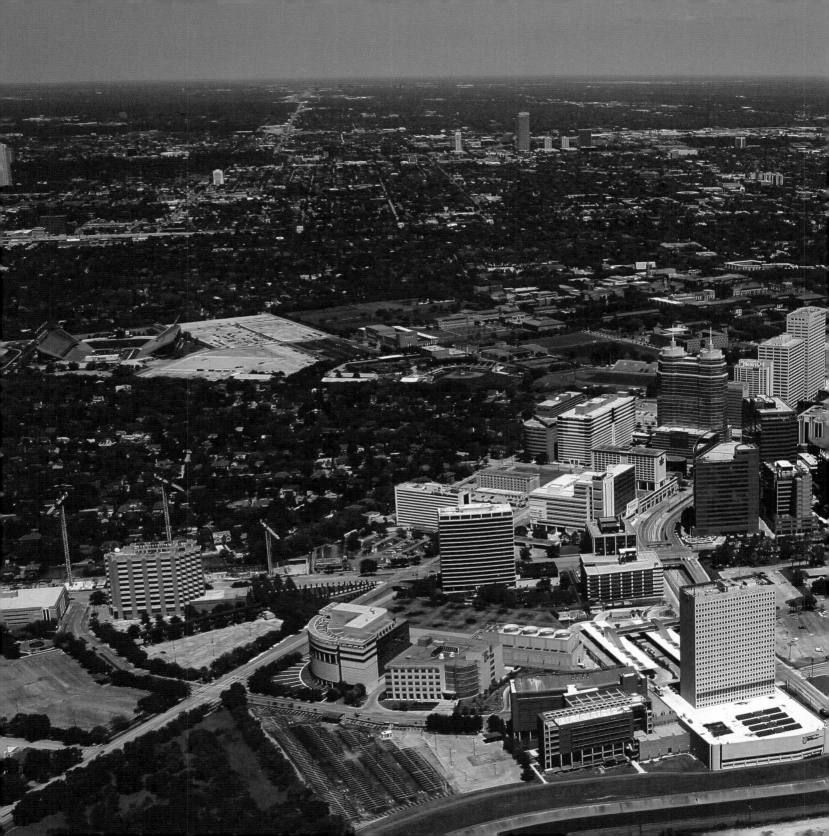

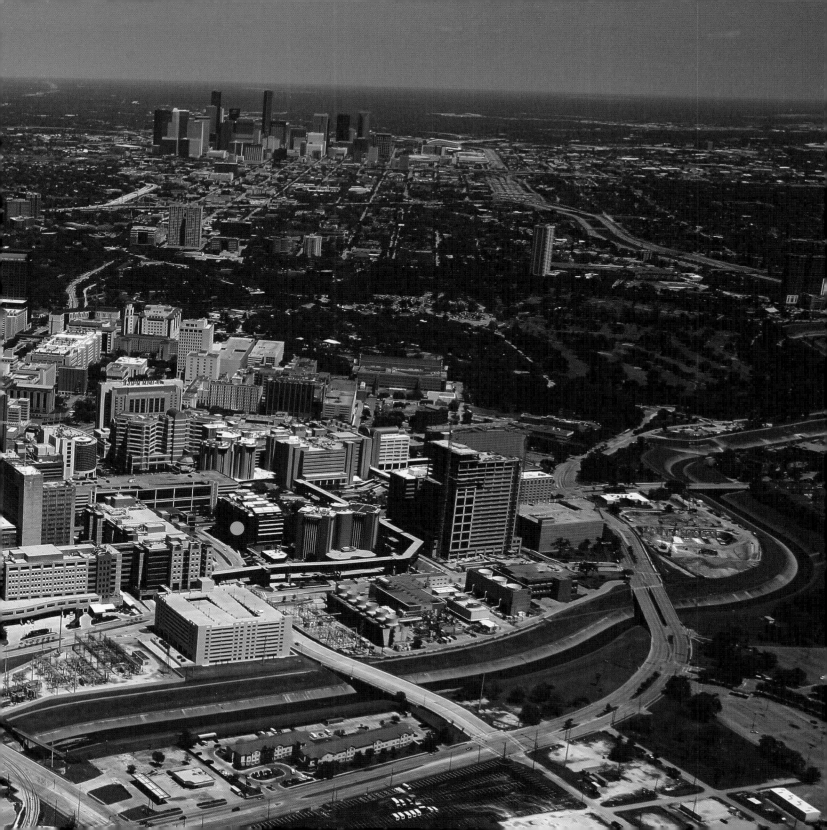

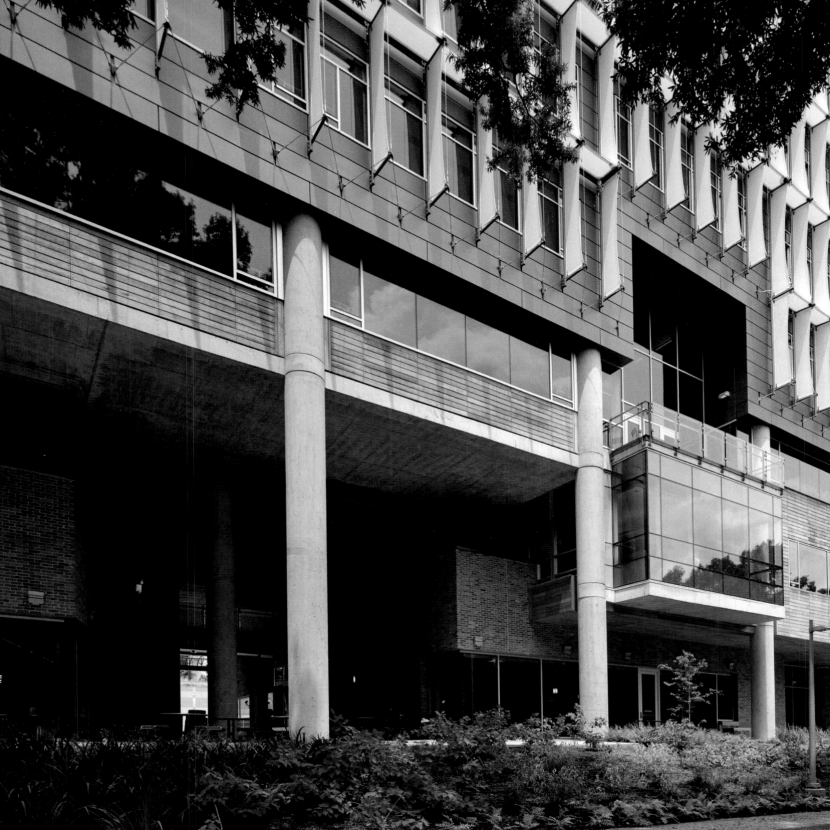

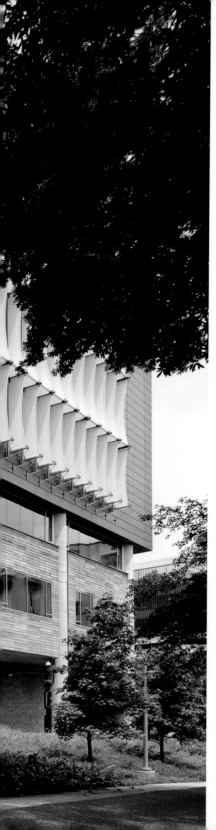

SITE

The University of Texas Health Science Center at Houston is located within the Texas Medical Center among the world's largest concentration of research and healthcare institutions. The site, a previously developed parcel within the dense urban environment of the Texas Medical Center, was challenging. The limited size, border restrictions and easements defined the general shape and confines of the building. The remaining buildable area dictated a less than ideal solar orientation, requiring the building's long façades to face due east and west, where they are open to exposure and unprotected from the harsh Houston sun.

The site is situated along the western edge of Grant Fay Park, one of the most beautiful amenities of the Medical Center, which profoundly influenced the design of the building and its site development. A variety of native species trees populate the park, creating a respite of shade, fragrant air and coolness. The UT School of Public Health sits directly to the southeast, forming the southern boundary of the park, and two major streets edge the site on the west and north. Both streets are flanked by Medical Center buildings and parking garages that provide limited contribution to the public realm and do not otherwise enhance the pedestrian experience.

The site conditions and constraints heavily influenced the building design and organization, which resulted in a building that is so deeply integrated with its site that its function is inextricably linked to its location.

LEFT
View from Grant Fay Park at east façade
and breezeway. East-facing glass is protected by
tensile fabric sunshade, recalling the nurturing
uniforms worn by nurses.

CONCEPTUAL STACKING DIAGRAM by floor

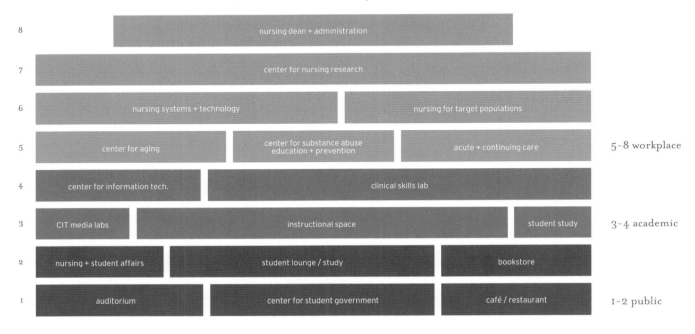

8	nursing dean + administration		
7	center for nursing research		
6	nursing systems + technology	nursing for target populations	
5	center for aging	center for substance abuse education + prevention	acute + continuing care
4	center for information tech.	clinical skills lab	
3	CIT media labs	instructional space	student study
2	nursing + student affairs	student lounge / study	bookstore
1	auditorium	center for student government	café / restaurant

5-8 workplace

3-4 academic

1-2 public

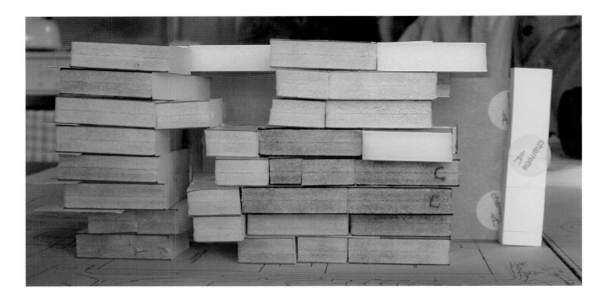

Conceptual Massing +
Program Model

oo4 PROGRAM

The design team began by analyzing the previously established program and comparing current and proposed utilization plans created by the School of Nursing. The program refinement revealed that the school would be better served by a slightly smaller building where the spaces were reorganized or shared to better support the activities and planned uses. By correctly sizing the program to support teaching, research and community, the design team more effectively balanced the needs of the greater community and the individual users, while also decreasing the building size and the construction cost. This also meant less square footage to maintain, less energy required for heating and cooling and a reduced environmental impact during construction and for the life of the building. To achieve a truly sustainable building, it was determined that the spaces must be occupied 80% of the time; therefore, academic scheduling was an important part of the programming process. The program—and subsequently, the building—became more sustainable before design commenced simply by determining that less was needed.

There are many nontraditional students in the nursing program, so the building program was adapted to provide study and support spaces to address these unique needs. Students are provided with comfortable study carrels overlooking the park, and the program includes other amenities such as a café and bookstore. During the design process, the Texas Legislature mandated increased enrollment in nursing schools statewide, increasing the Full Time Equivalent (FTE) for the new building by 20%. The balance established with the revised program meant that the facility could successfully fulfill its dual role: community spaces could serve the entire Texas Medical Center population, while the UT School of Nursing could be served by its required, dedicated spaces.

The separation and organization of the three main types of space contained in the building—public, academic and workplace—is supported by the idea of a vertical campus. Three vertically stacked zones of space provide a clear organization for the various types of academic environments.

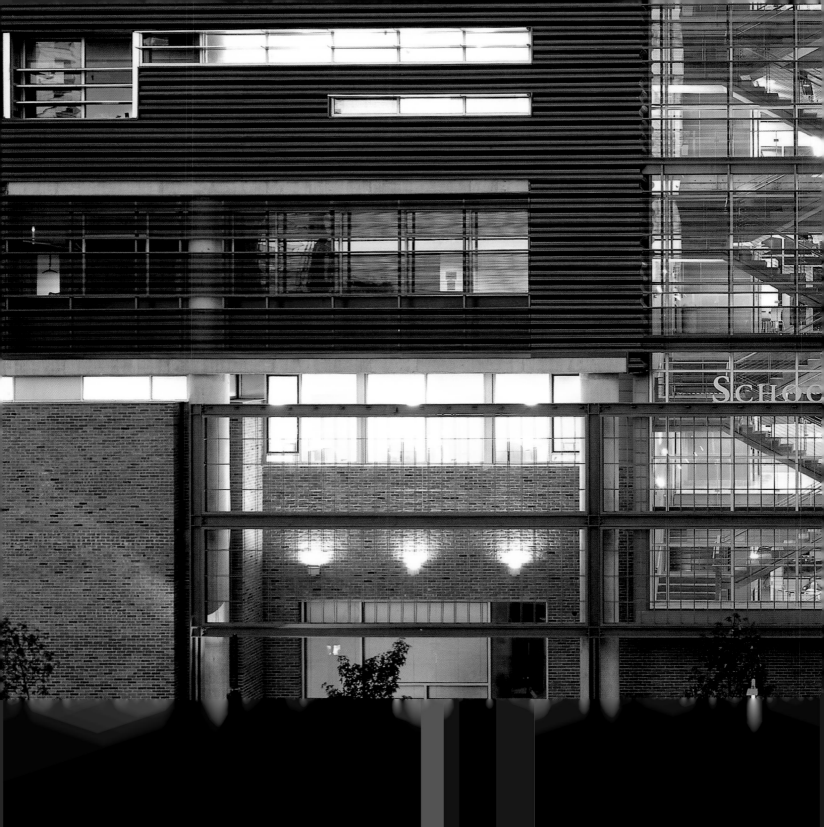

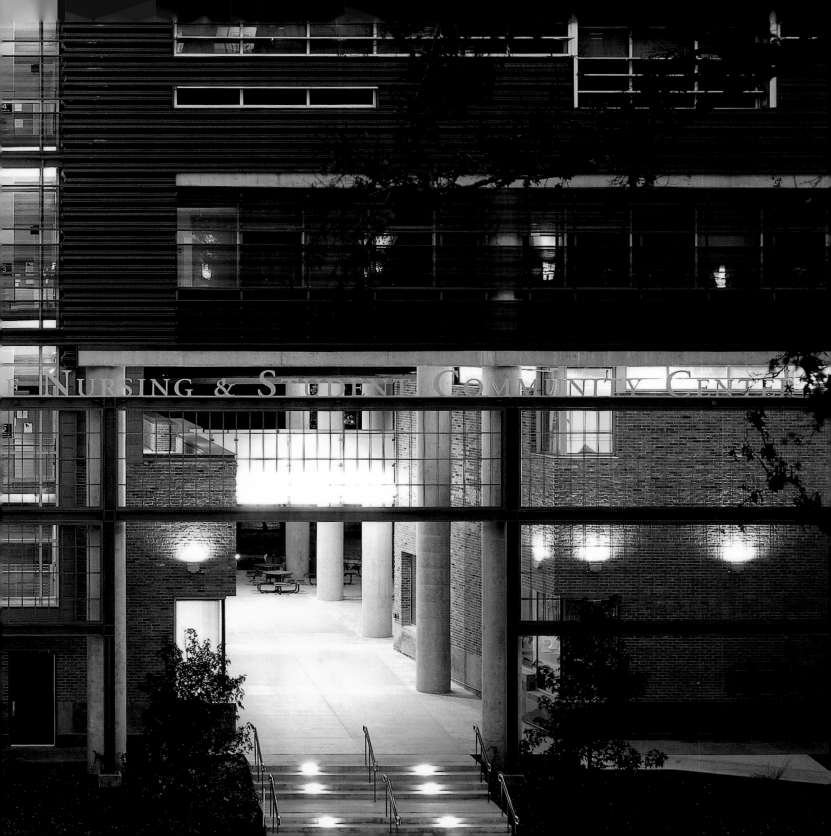

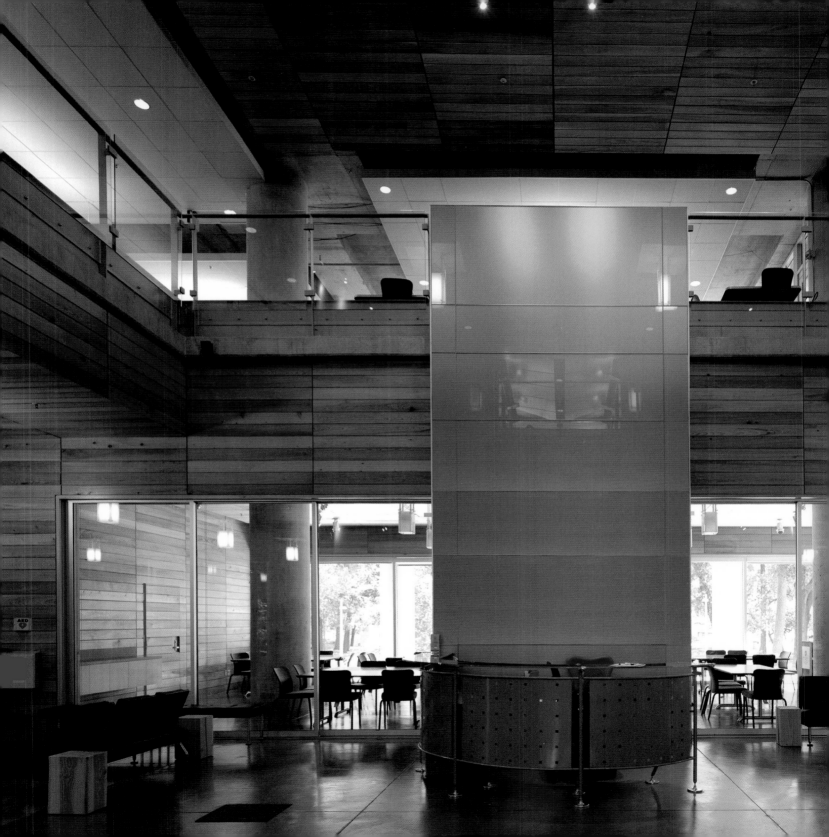

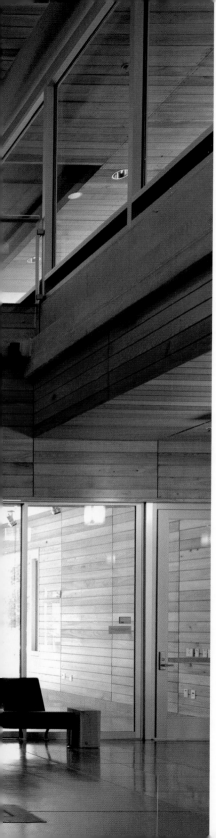

LEFT
Two-story lobby unites reception area
with student community services. Materials
such as exposed concrete floor, salvaged
cypress walls and ceilings and copper glass
partition warm the space.

OVERLEAF
Two-story café and bookstore with views to
breezeway and main building entrance.

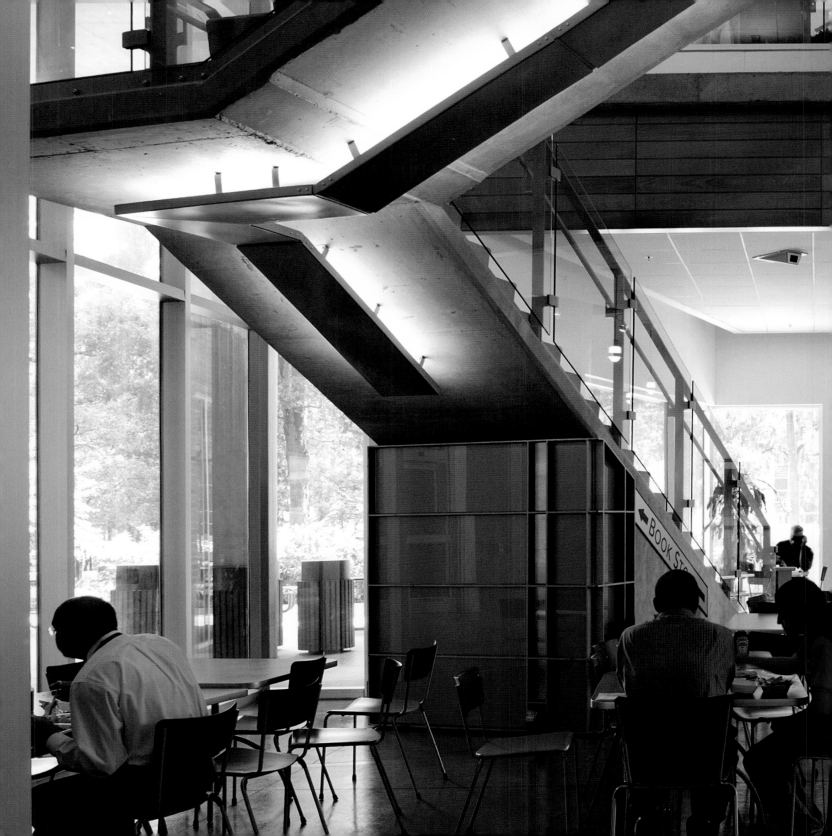

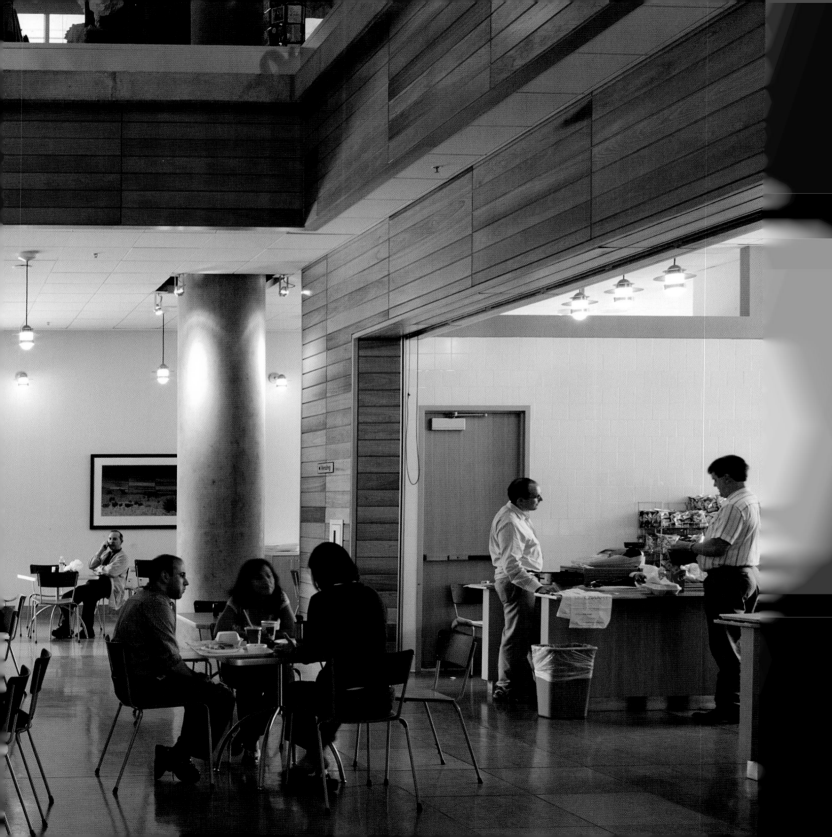

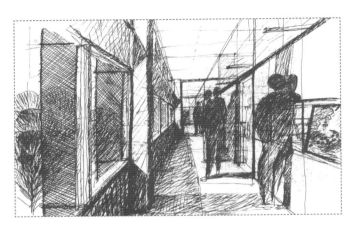
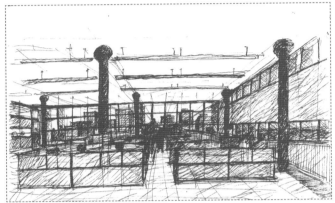
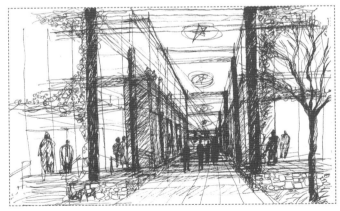
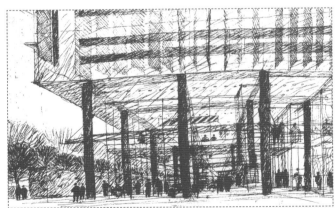

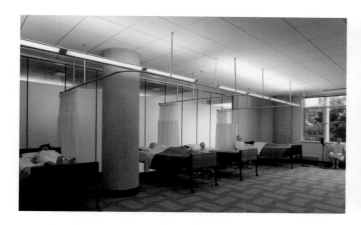
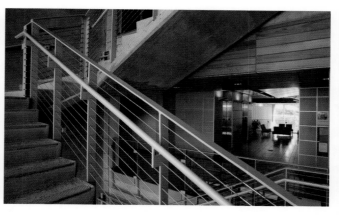
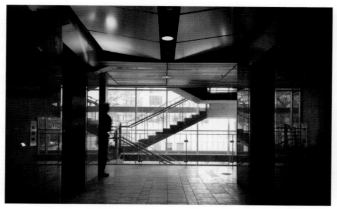
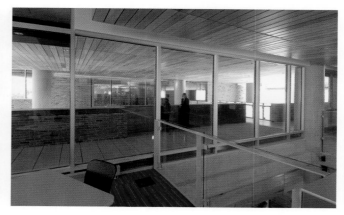

CLOCKWISE FROM TOP LEFT
Clinical-skills labs. Centrally located stair encourages use.
Daylight and access to views were enlisted at every opportunity.
Student Community Center with views to breezeway.

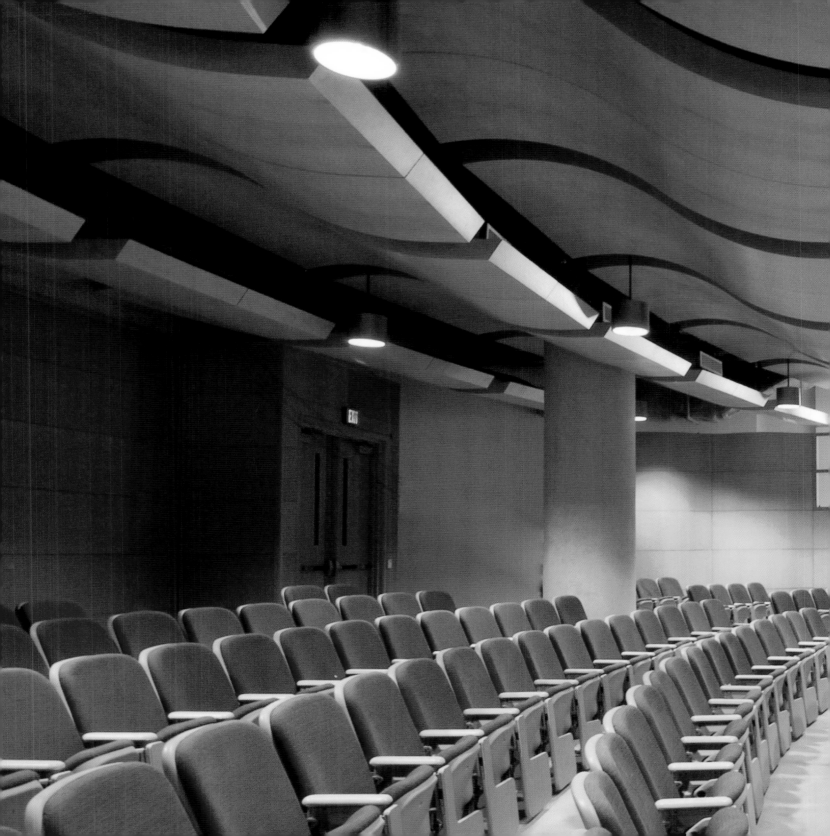

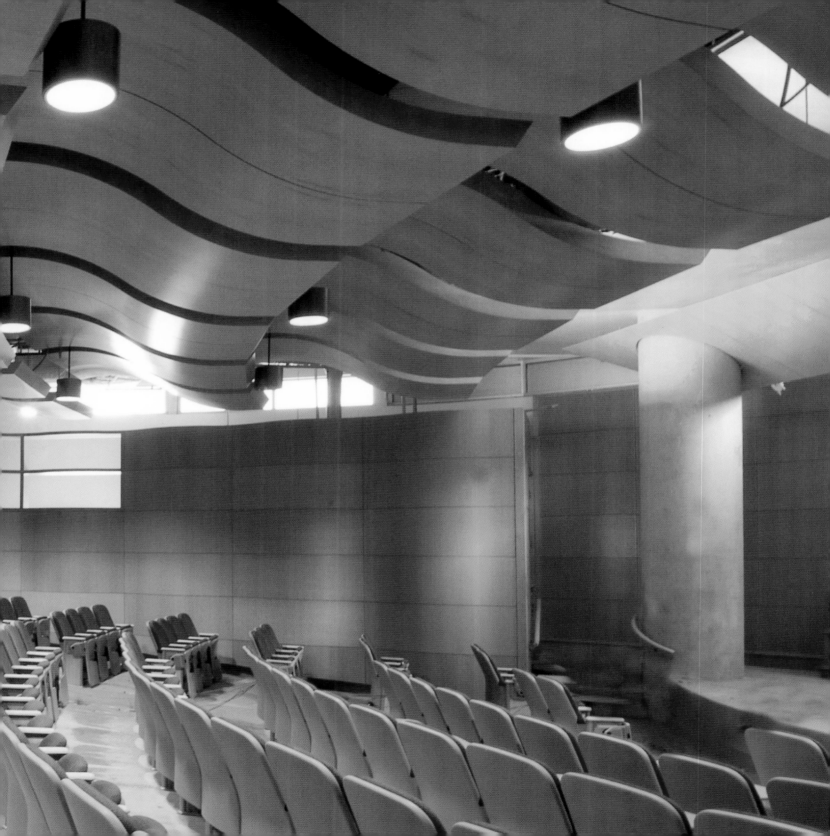

005 DESIGN CONCEPT

The concept for this building is rooted in the practice of professional nursing—both the nurturing aspect of nursing care and the idea of perpetuating health. The building is simultaneously sheltering, nurturing and healing. It was designed to communicate, interact, teach and provide inspiration to students, staff and the larger community.

With straightforward, authentic and transparent design, the School of Nursing and Student Community Center is intended to establish benchmarks for healthy buildings, daylight, visual acuity, cognitive learning, pedagogy and the capacity to learn and collaborate. Flexibility, durability and reduced operating costs were all foundations of the design methodology.

The plan and section were conceived jointly to create a building that responds to the site and program by organizing building functions to maximize exposure to the adjacent park, views and daylight. Carved spaces penetrate the building—such as a breezeway, horizontal atrium and three vertical atria—to introduce light and connect the building to its site and environment.

The plan is a simple rectangle reflecting the allowable area for building, which is further organized into two zones on each floor. The eastern three quarters house offices, classrooms, laboratories, the auditorium, a bookstore, café and other primary spaces. The western zone is primarily a service zone reserved for conference rooms, support spaces and secondary offices and laboratories. The building design places the public spaces in a desirable location along the east edge near the park. With the vertical circulation and mechanical core set to the west, the maximum open area faces the east, where park views and daylight enhance the spatial quality. This larger eastern zone also allows flexibility and can be more easily transformed as uses change over time.

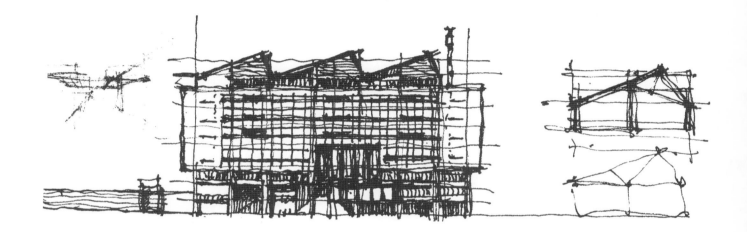

ABOVE
Early concept sketch showing the
development of the unique roof profile
and façade design.

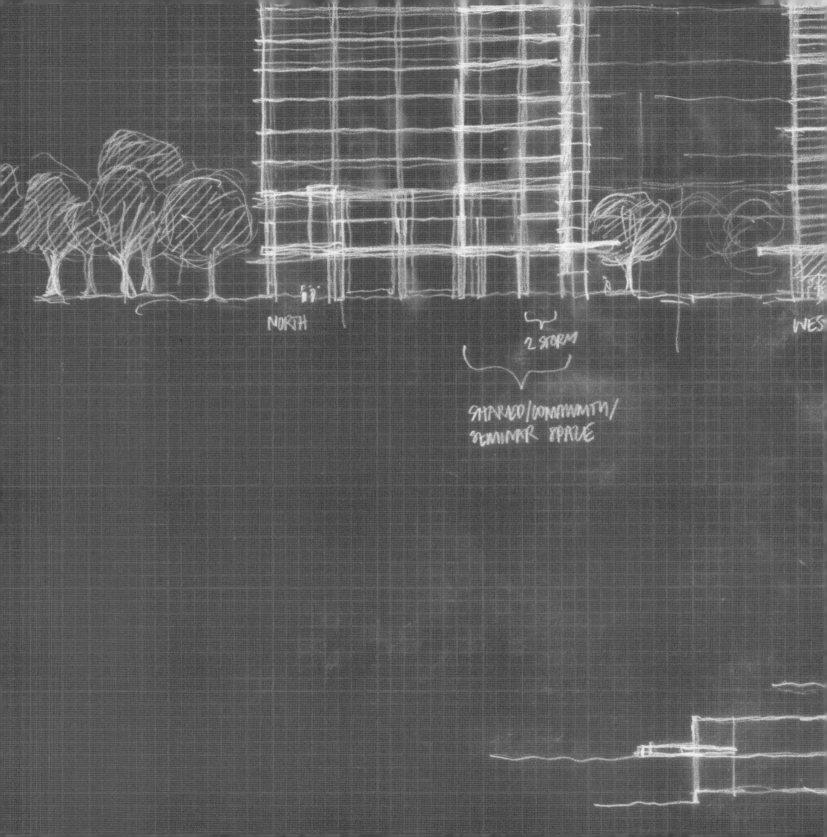

NORTH

2 STORM

SHARED/COMMUNITY/
SEMINAR SPACE

WES

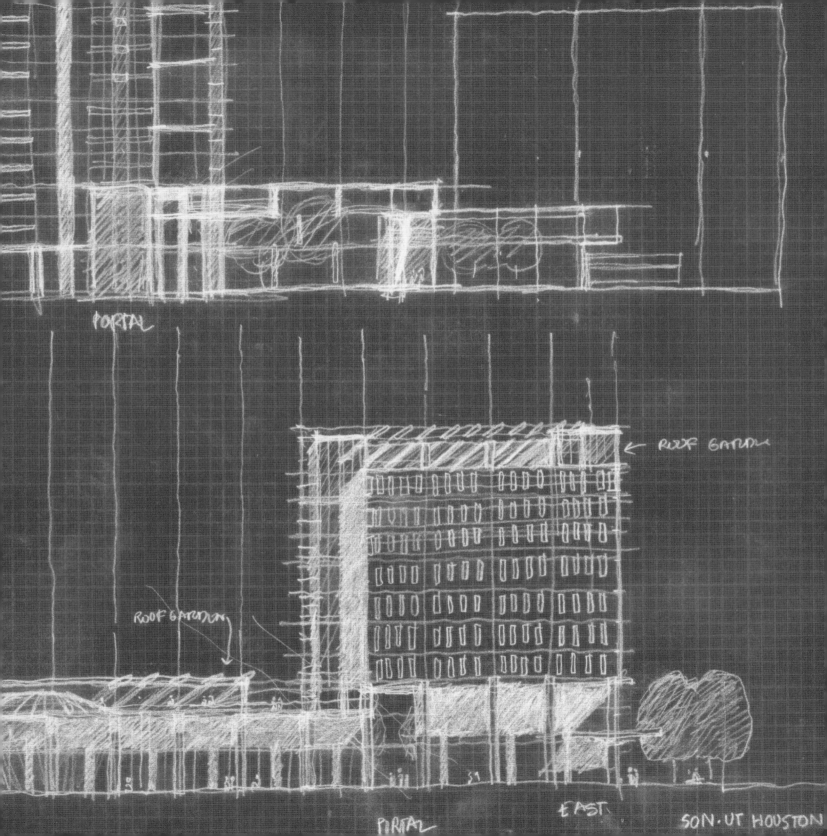

PORTAL

ROOF GARDEN

ROOF GARDEN

PORTAL

EAST

SON·UT HOUSTON

The section is further organized and articulated by three spaces that connect the building to its site and environment, deliver daylight deep into the building and organize the building into a vertical campus. A breezeway, or dog run, bisects the lower two floors and connects Bertner Avenue to the west and Grant Fay Park to the east, serving as a literal and symbolic gateway for the building. The ground floor and second floor are reserved for the most interactive community spaces—the auditorium, café, student services, bookstore, gathering spaces and other student- and faculty-centered uses. The breezeway intersects these levels with seductive views of the park and provides a shaded, open-air entry and gathering place. On the second level, an outdoor walkway crosses the breezeway, and perimeter porches encourage outdoor circulation. A direct visual connection to the UT School of Public Health strengthens the greater campus fabric.

Floors three and four are the primary academic spaces—classrooms, practical laboratories, patient rooms and other learning environments. A two-story horizontal atrium captures and introduces eastern light into the building while connecting the space to the park beyond.

The top four floors—levels five through eight—house the faculty and graduate student offices and research laboratories. These floors share three atria topped with sky-lights that are ringed with offices and workspaces. The space utilizes demountable, moveable partitions to maintain flexibility and delineate work space.

Just as the inside of the building is designed to be a productive and uplifting environment for teaching the next generation of nurturers, the site has its own therapeutic aspects. In addition to the lush and tranquil park, gardens and a stone labyrinth offer opportunities for healing meditation and contemplation.

RIGHT
A horizontal atrium links the academic
floors with a two-story space that overlooks
Grant Fay Park.

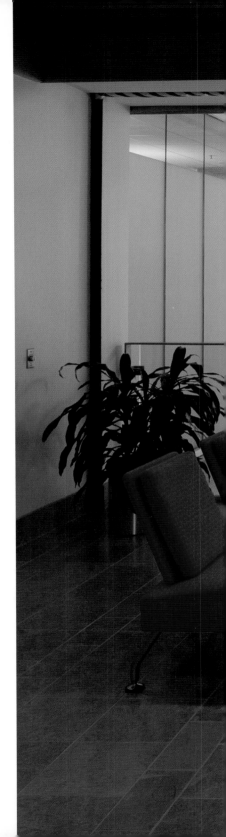

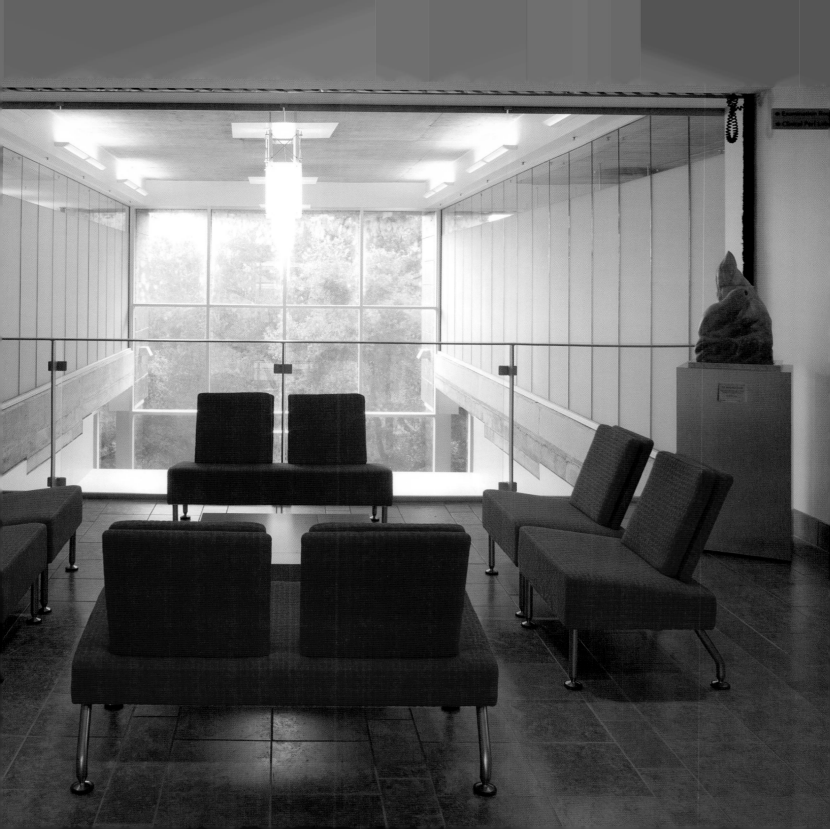

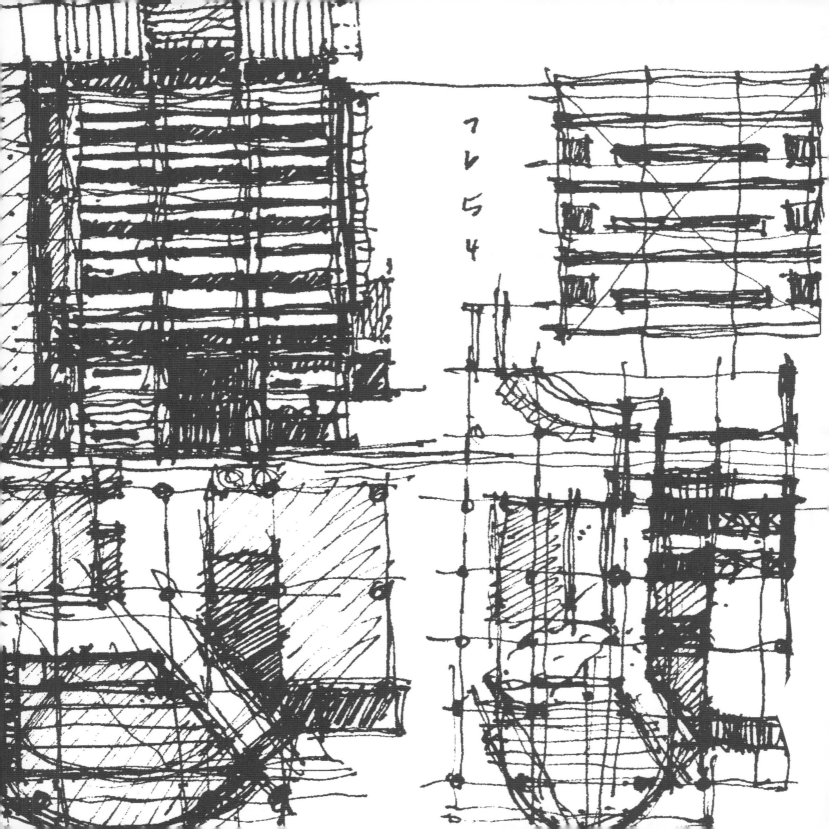

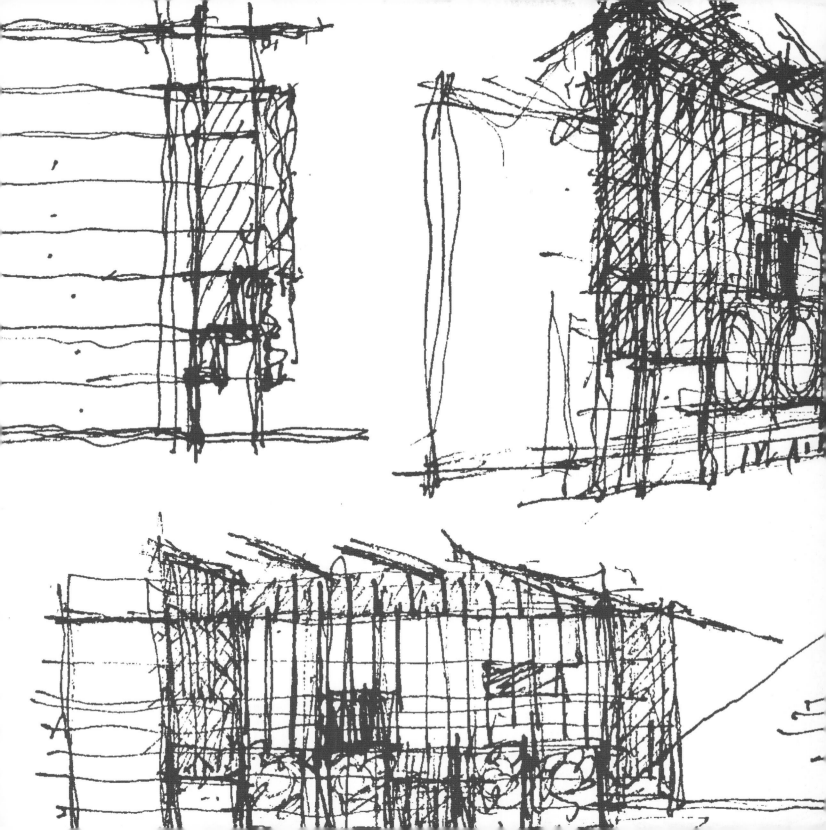

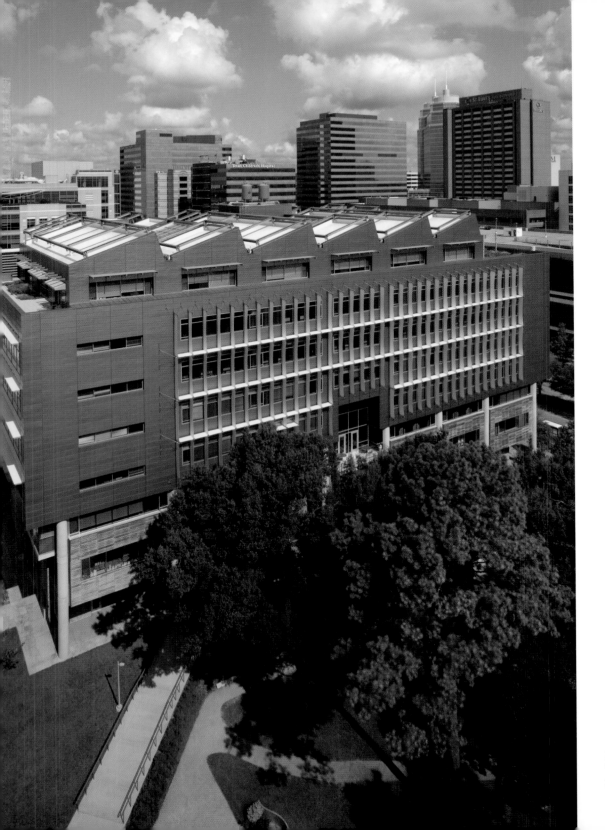

LEFT
View from Grant Fay Park
looking west.

oo6 ENVELOPE DESIGN CONCEPT :
FIVE FAÇADES

Due to site orientation, harsh environmental conditions and program requirements, each of the four elevations and the roof, or fifth façade, reflect the unique conditions of each exposure. Each of the five façades has individually tailored fenestration and sun control to increase the quality and effectiveness of daylight while simultaneously rejecting unwanted heat. The result is a facility that tells the story of the sun's path.

In order to effectively utilize daylight at the building's perimeter, daylight modeling and analysis informed the exact placement and sizing of window openings. Sophisticated envelope design informed the percentage of glazing selected for each façade. The design analysis specified glazing with specific properties based on application: low-e coatings, low u-value, spectrally selective shading devices and light-reflecting devices.

The need to reduce cooling loads is expressed through shading devices, rooftop design and covered outdoor spaces that *minimize* heat gain and glare.

The building organization responds to the path of the sun by placing critical functions in a way that avoids the penetration of direct light, heat and glare, providing for a more comfortable environment.

Adjacent buildings and the landscape also inform the building's shade patterns. On the upper levels of the south and west façades, aluminum light shelves reflect daylight and reduce glare, and on the east façade, translucent sailcloth fins and light shelves do the same. On the lower levels, the leafy canopy in the park shades the building. The breezeway naturally cools the outdoor space by harnessing the venturi effect and the cooler ambient temperatures of the park to the east.

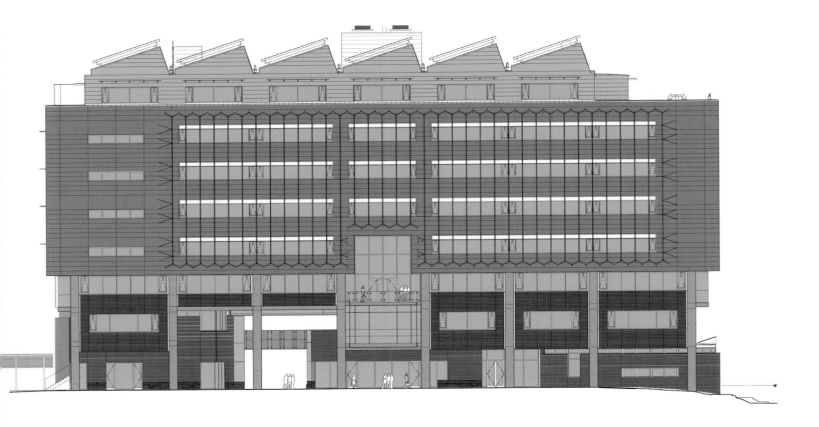

The building's vertical organization and fenestration are interrelated. Tactile materials, such as recycled brick, granite and sinker cypress siding parallel the public usage of the lowest two levels; and durable, efficient materials clad the upper six levels as building functions become more private and the protective skin must resist the environmental forces of the climate. The aluminum curtain wall of these levels—with 92% recycled content—is modeled on rainscreen design and has a high-performance vapor barrier, as well as a highly insulated wall section (>R30). This rainscreen panel system employs a water barrier and a three-inch air space behind the aluminum panels. This acts as a double skin in the hot Texas climate.

The building's envelope contributes greatly to the overall sustainability of the facility and to all six categories used to evaluate buildings in the Leadership in Energy and Environmental Design (LEED®) process. In the preliminary analysis, the roof was as important as the façade design. Plantings, along with green-roof technology, enhance the portions of the roof accessible from the office areas. The roof itself has a high-performance profile: it is designed for the addition of photovoltaic panels and has a high reflectivity, low emissivity membrane roof and a highly insulated roof section. The sawtooth roof creates a unique profile within the Texas Medical Center.

LEFT
Material investigation drawing at east elevation:
at the entry level of the building, the materials are
tactile and scaled to the human touch; as the
building rises, materials become tougher and more
impervious to weather and exposure.

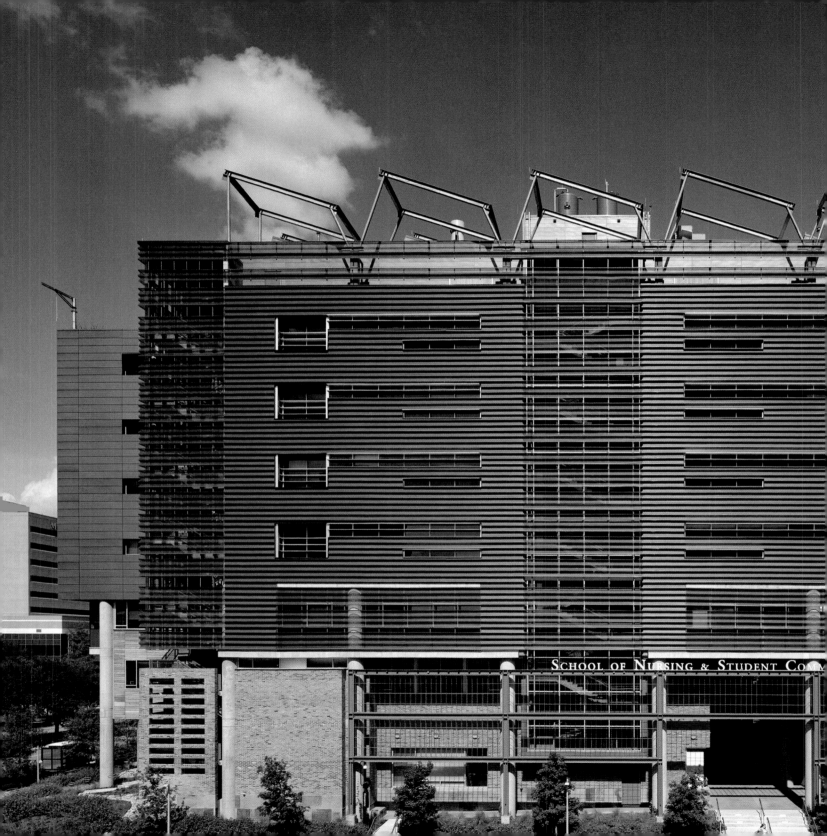

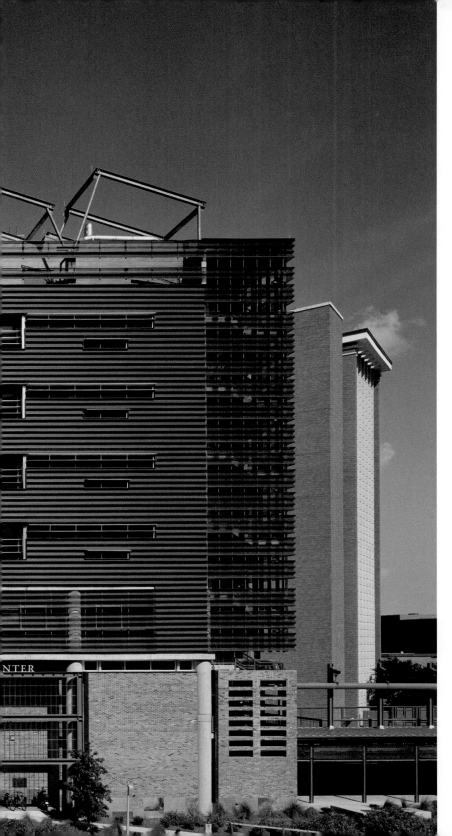

LEFT
West elevation: Glazed area is 22% of the surface.
Perforated aluminum panels shade the central stair on
both sides. Light shelves provide shade and bounce
light into seminar rooms. Primary materials include
salvaged brick base, recycled aluminum siding
(80% by content) and recycled aluminum window
frames (90% by content).

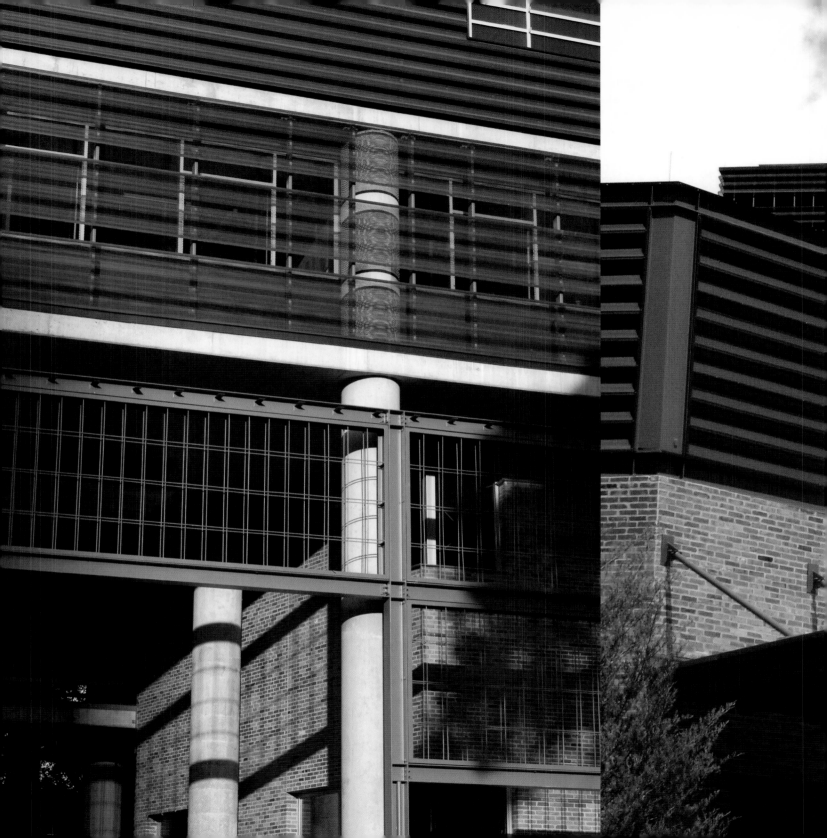

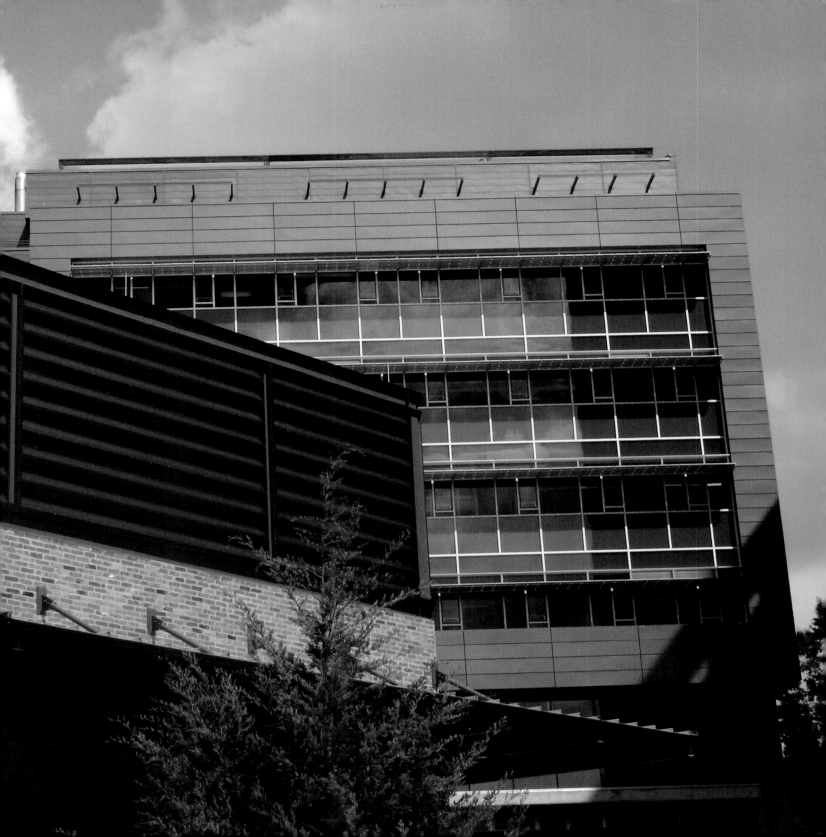

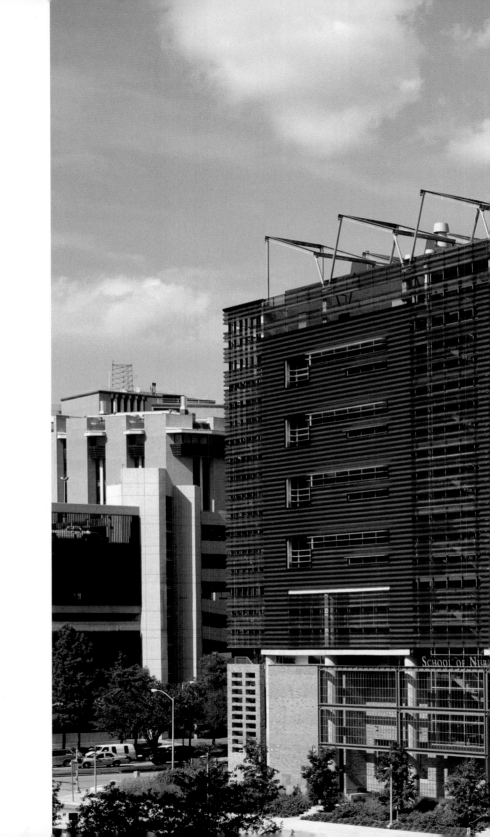

RIGHT
View from southwest shows the
School of Nursing sited at a
prominent campus intersection.

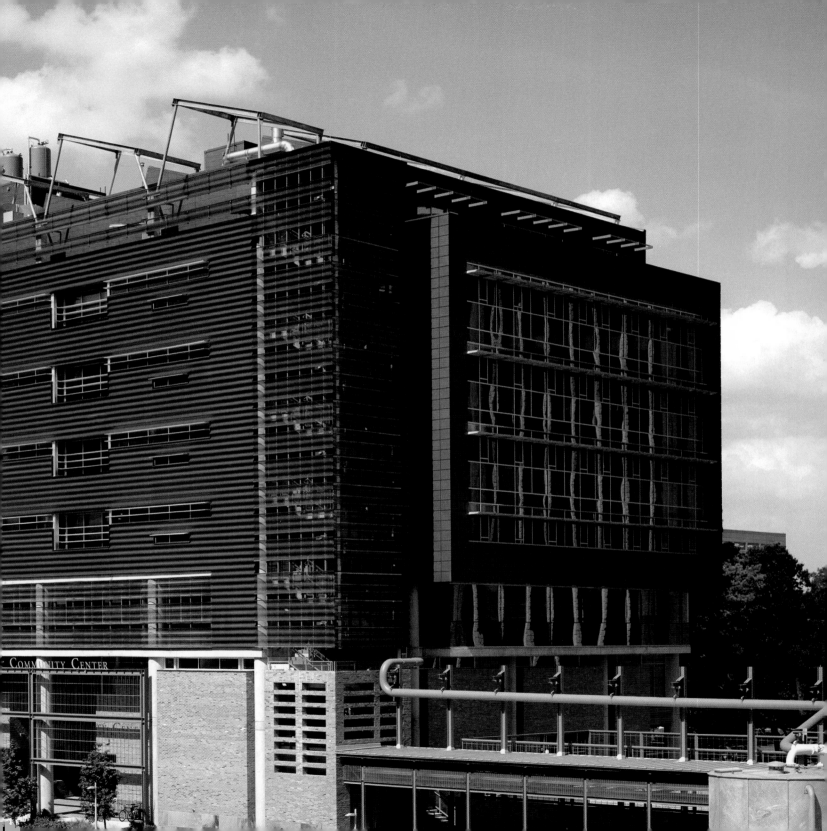

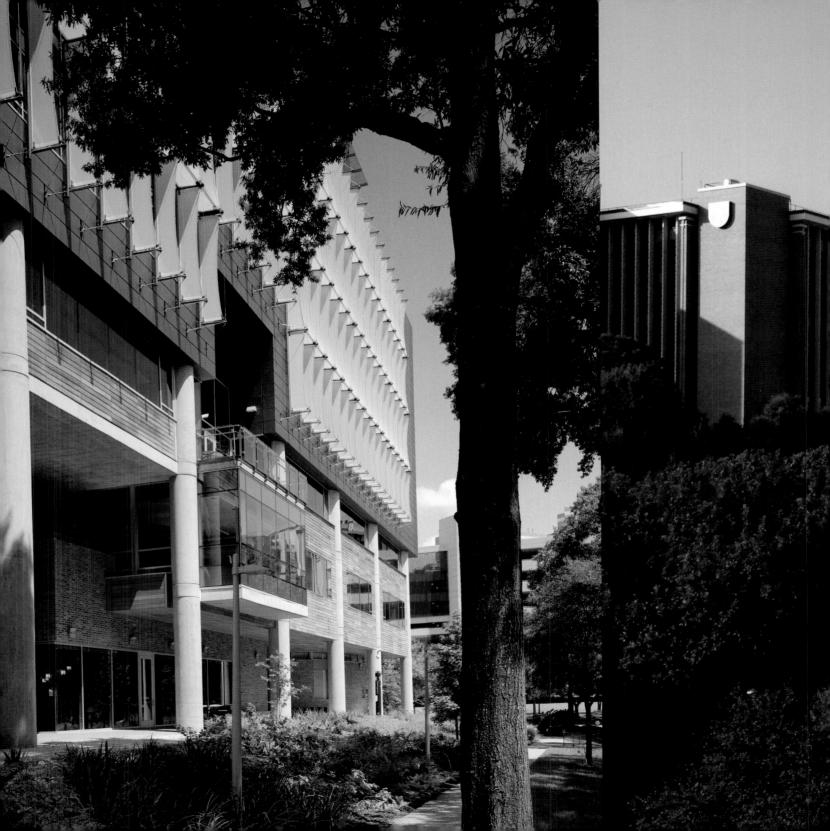

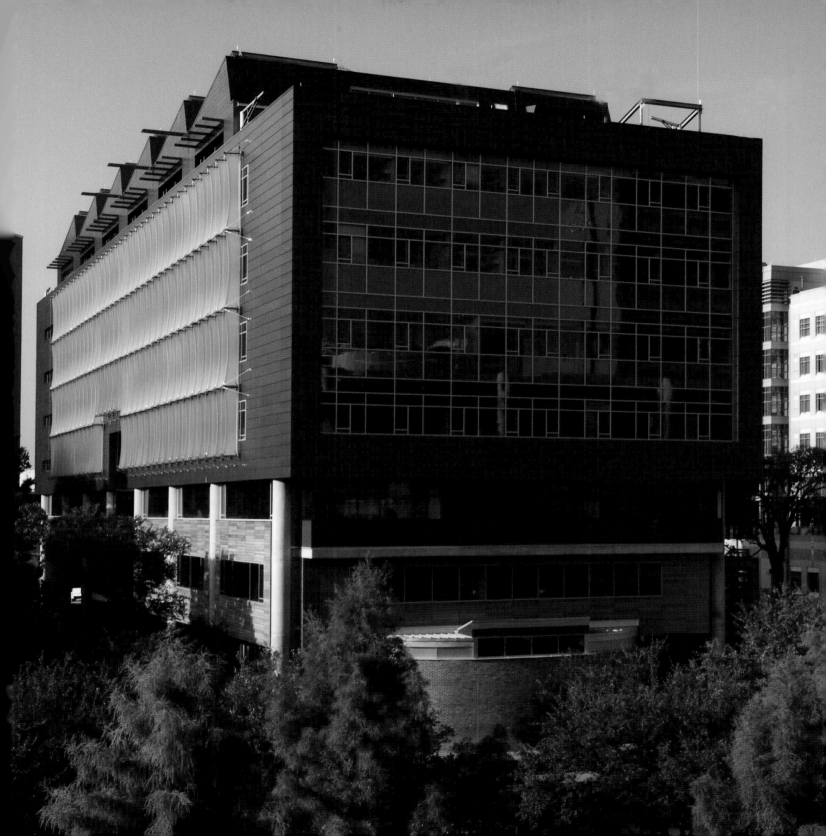

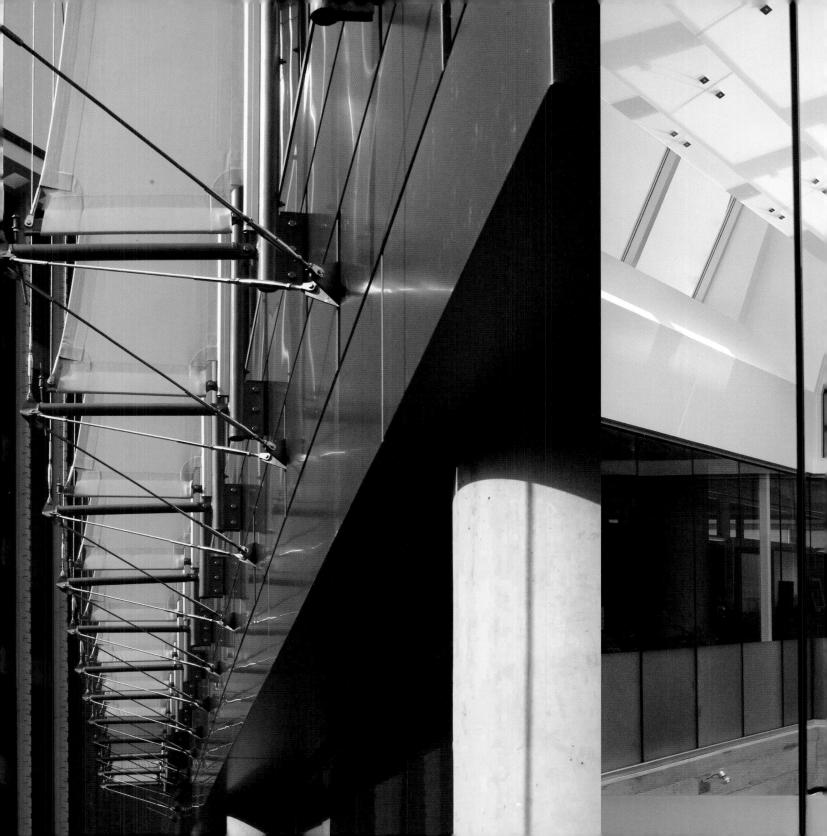

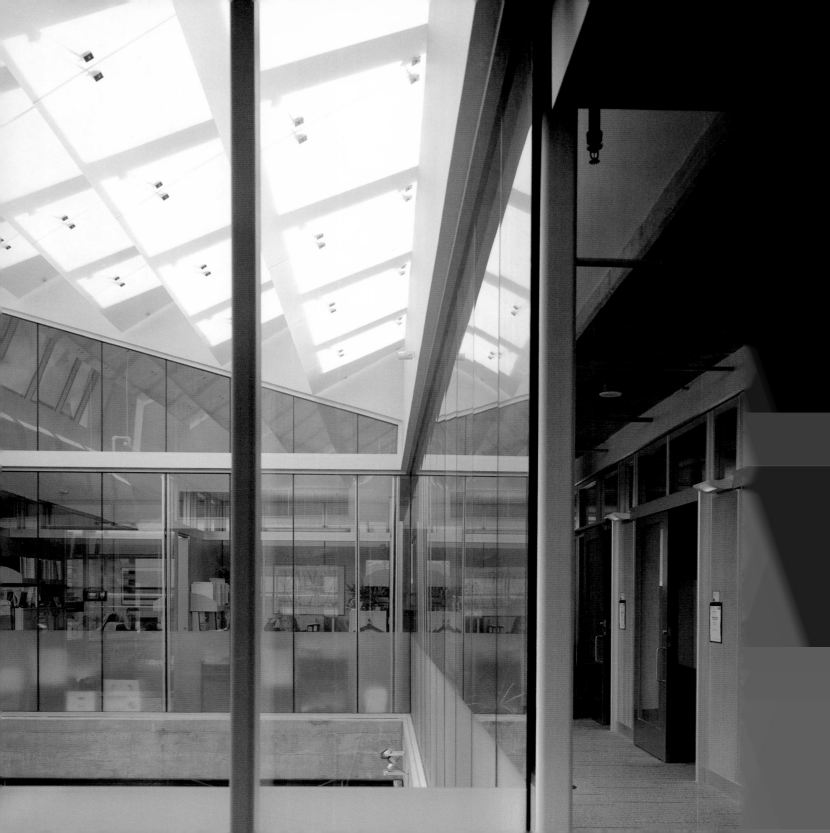

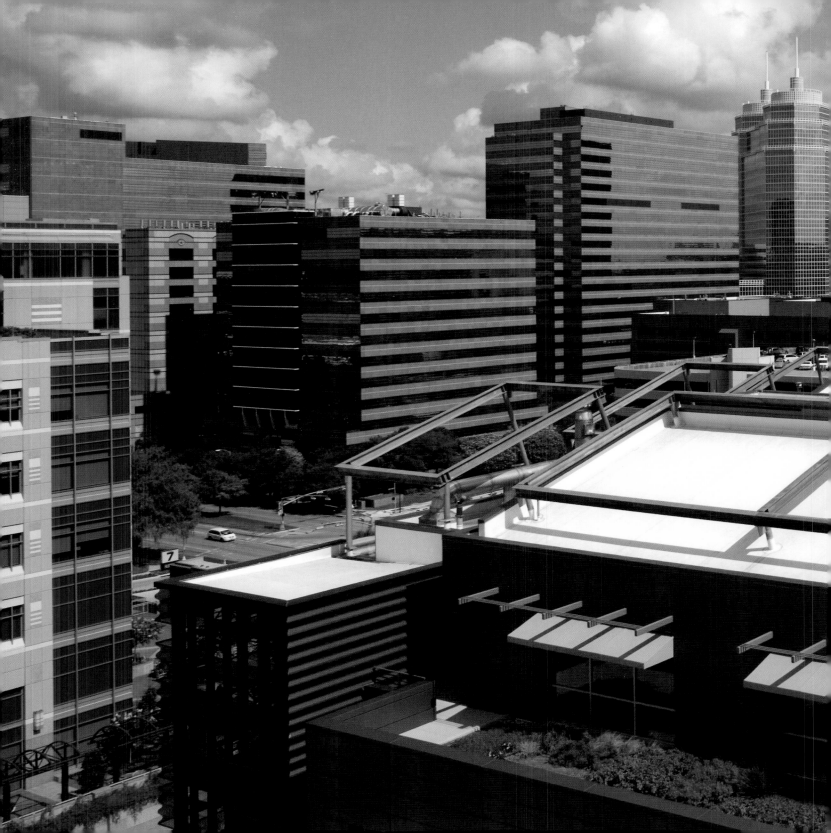

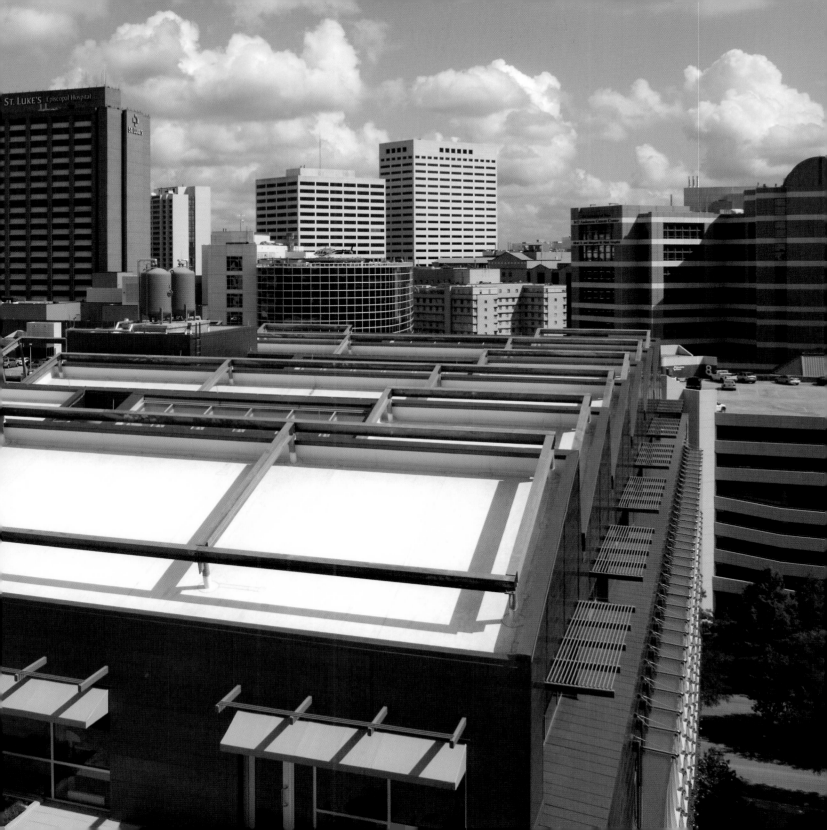

007 DAYLIGHTING DESIGN :
A PROCESS OF INTUITIVE + SCIENTIFIC DESIGN

The team designed the building to maximize daylighting and access to views for all occupants. A strong organizational concept for the plan and section of the facility drove the daylighting strategies, and the concept evolved to include more interrelated building systems as different design tactics were refined for each of the five façades. Initially, the team studied alternatives for introducing controlled light into the building without modeling or engineering input.

The early *intuitive* studies proposed that daylit penetrations would carry light deep into the building and connect interior spaces, emphasizing the idea of a vertical campus and the connection with Grant Fay Park.

Energy and daylight modeling tools were then employed to test these intuitive ideas and truly understand the conditions. This allowed the team to design the most effective systems for windows, skylights, shading systems, electric lighting systems and other elements. Each of the alternative design schemes was simulated through a yearly cycle to fully understand each of the approaches and its benefits. The measurements from these simulations were then compared so that definitive, scientific decisions could be made about using specific strategies for light quality, quantity, energy performance, costs and life-cycle criteria.

The scientific process allowed the design team to articulate the daylighting strategies for this visionary educational environment, and the result has intangible yet appreciable benefits. The cohesive strategies include an integrated façade design, vertical atria and a horizontal atrium to provide controlled daylight. The visual connection to the outdoors boosts productivity and reduces absenteeism, increased learning occurs due to better mental function and increased visual acuity and the university benefits from energy savings.

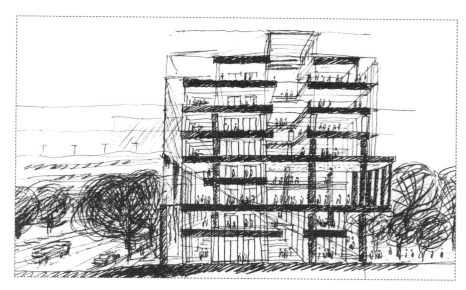

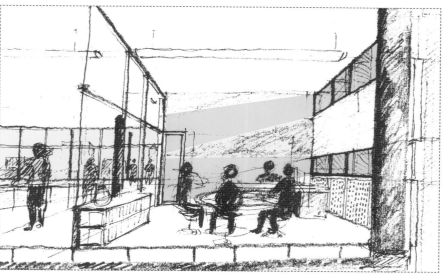

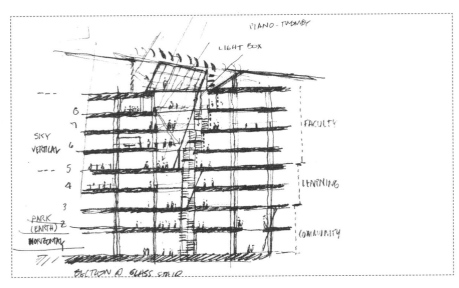

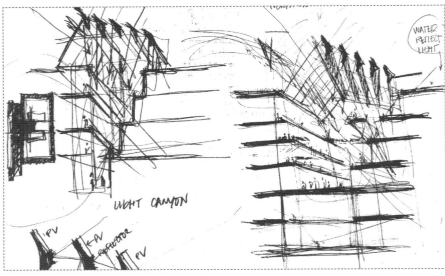

LEFT
Concept sketches showing the
intuitive development of the atria.

RIGHT
Radiance images showing the
scientific development of the atria
utilizing computer modeling.

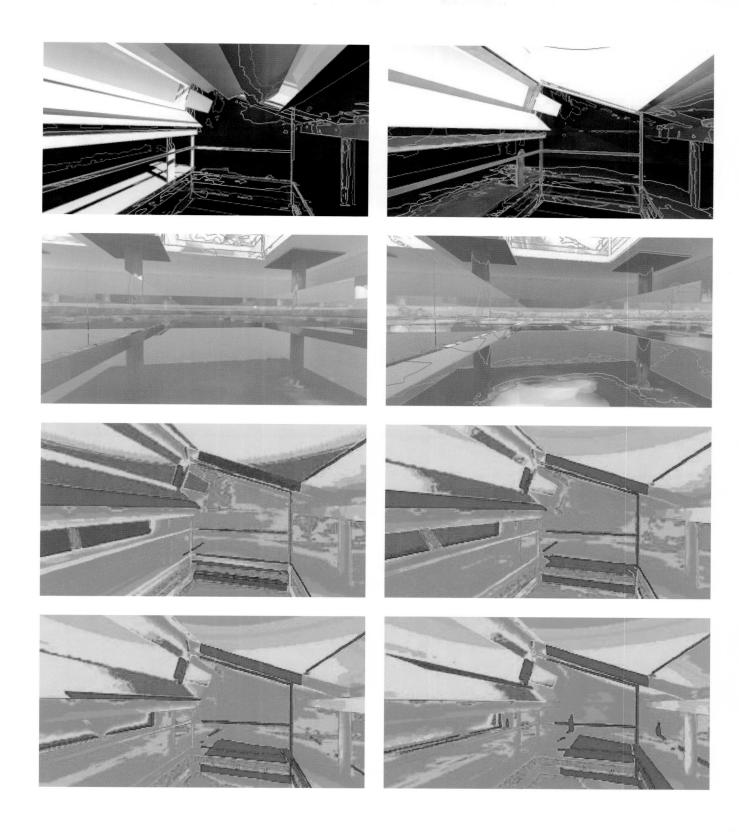

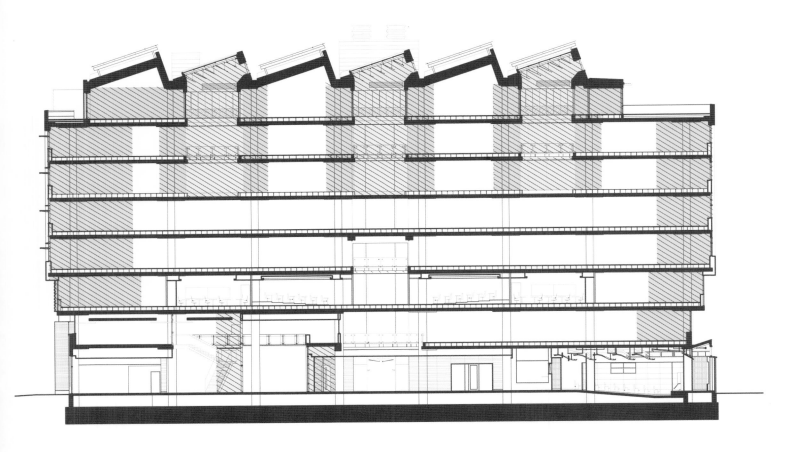

ABOVE + OPPOSITE
Diagrams demonstrate daylight
penetration into the building.

0 5 10   20

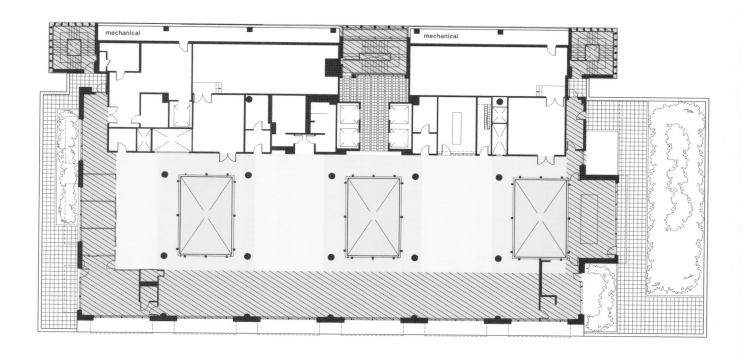

mechanical

mechanical

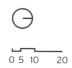

0 5 10 20

OVERLEAF
The atrium was sized
based on computer modeling.

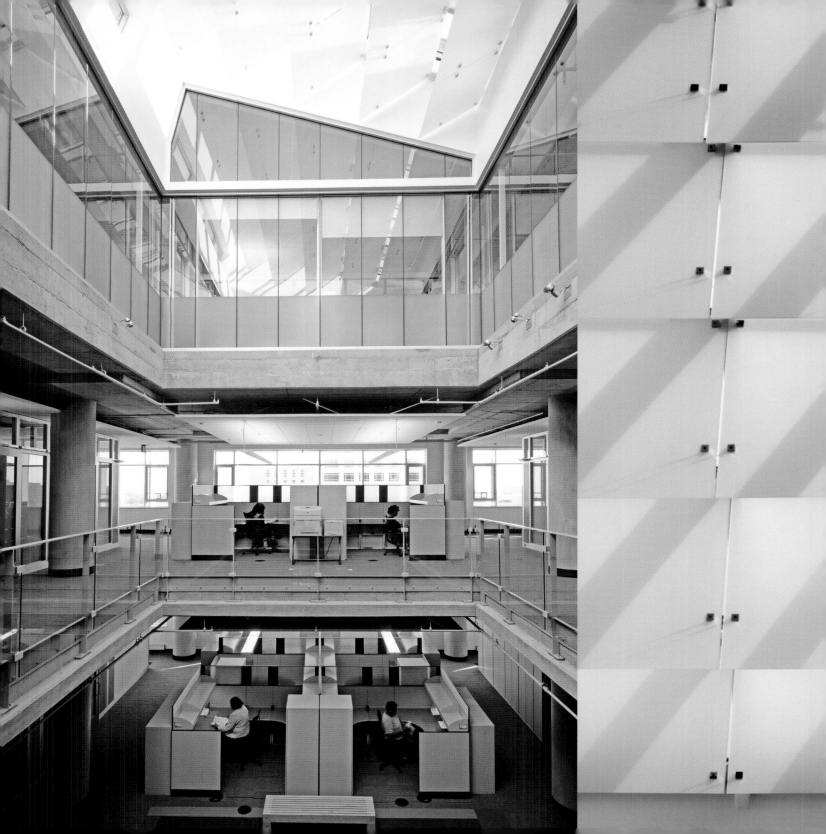

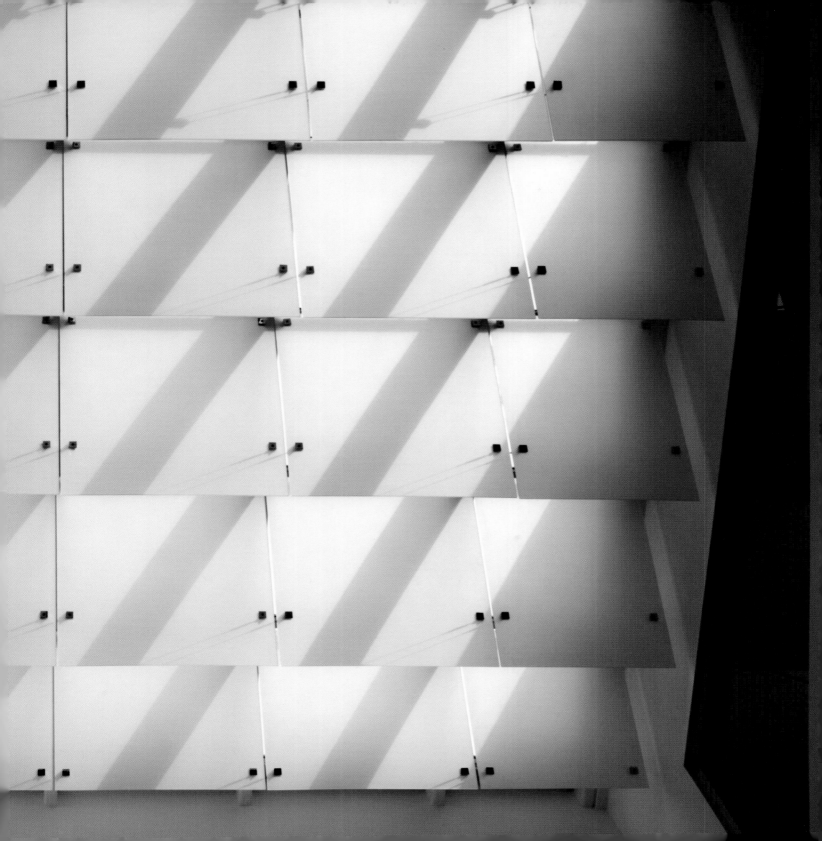

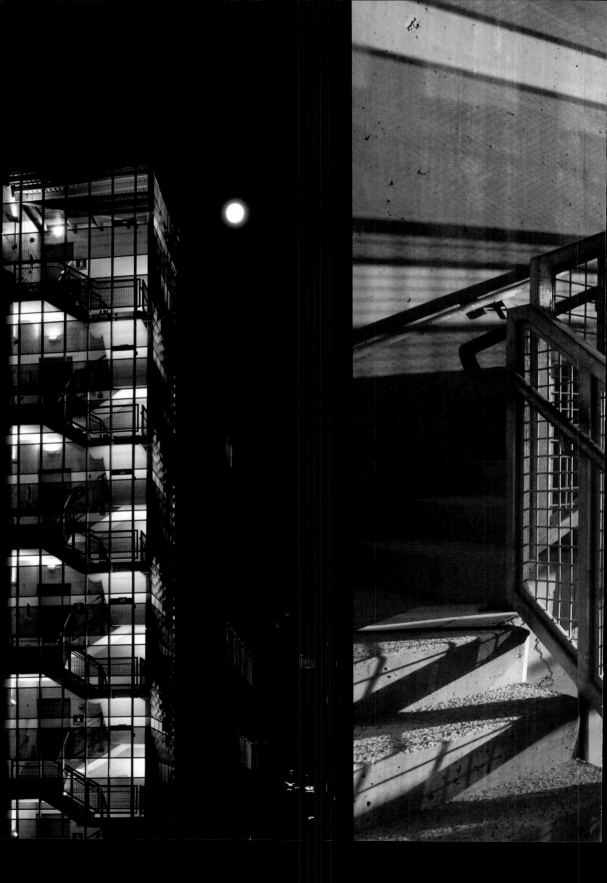

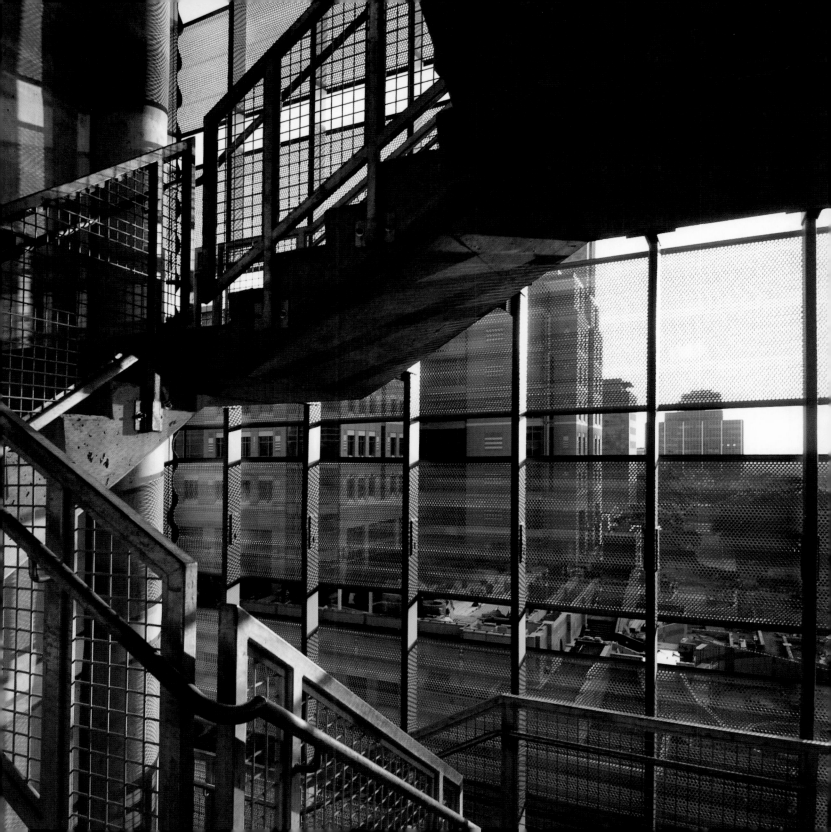

oo8 SUSTAINABLE DESIGN STRATEGIES

The team was challenged to achieve a LEED® Gold or Platinum rating, based on the U.S. Green Building Council's LEED certification program. This directive also required that the design be accomplished with no more than a 5% up-front cost premium over similar University of Texas System projects. It was immediately apparent that a highly integrated design was necessary to meet the challenges and achieve these goals.

The six categories of sustainable design, as identified in LEED, served as the general outline for the approach that the team followed in documenting the sustainable design strategies of the project:

1 SUSTAINABLE SITES
2 WATER EFFICIENCY
3 INDOOR ENVIRONMENTAL QUALITY
4 ENERGY + ATMOSPHERE
5 MATERIALS + RESOURCES
6 INNOVATION + DESIGN PROCESS

I. SUSTAINABLE SITES

The sustainable site design strategies for the project included reducing the heat island effect by limiting paved area and utilizing green roofs on the building wherever possible. Light trespass is reduced from the building site by the careful placement of directed and shielded outdoor light fixtures and an overall reduction in the use of exterior illumination.

The building occupies almost the entire available site within the dense campus environment and was constructed over an existing building site; the previous building was deconstructed by the university as phase one of the new construction project. The team responded to the building's siting adjacent to Grant Fay Park, by crafting a landscape and ecological design that enhances the experience of visitors to the park. Because of the limited parameters of the site, the roof represents a majority of the site surface area. To address runoff, portions of the roof were designed as green roofs, and the balance of the roof area mitigates heat gain through its design.

The architectural design of the school encourages users to enter the landscape. The double-height breezeway is cool and shaded, even during the hottest Houston days. An elevated walkway bridges the breezeway and connects to second-level balconies that are nestled into the trees. Spaces located adjacent to the park,including the auditorium, take advantage of the daylight and views.

Establishing inviting outdoor spaces was key to the site development. A meditative labyrinth adjacent to the facility enhances the presence of the adjacent park. The local ecology is very important to the UT School of Nursing. Trees in the park to the east of the building provide critical shade, and onsite landscaping and plant materials also play an important role. The team worked with the university's urban forester to select and specify indigenous species for planted areas. These plantings are irrigated by rainwater that is harvested and stored on site and require very little maintenance.

OVERLEAF
The breezeway's cool and shaded cover shelters the main entry and walkway that joins the second floor with the café and bookstore.

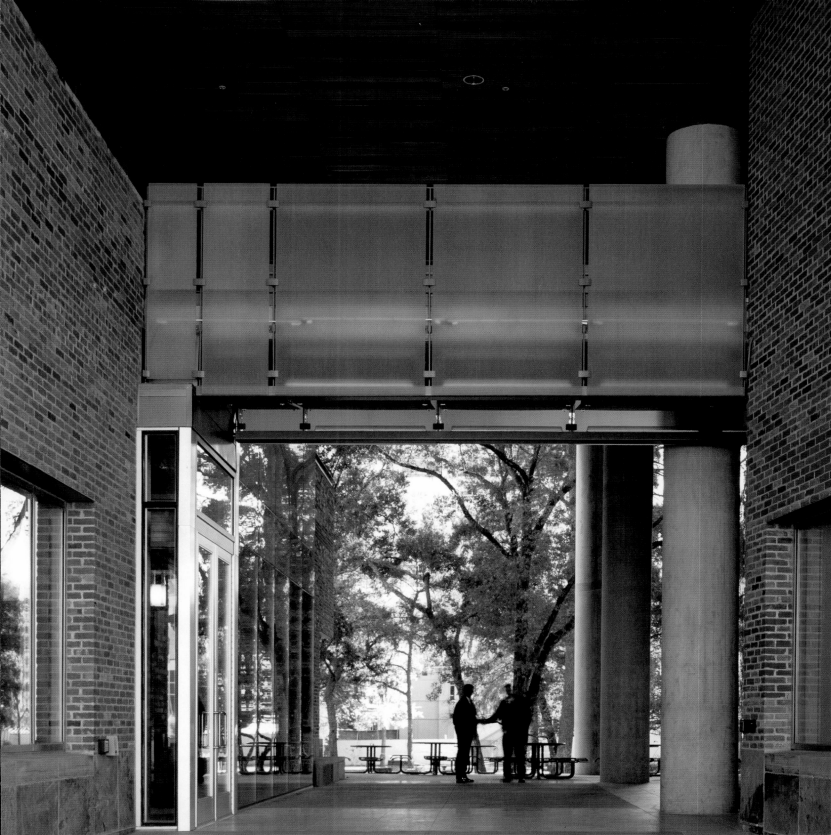

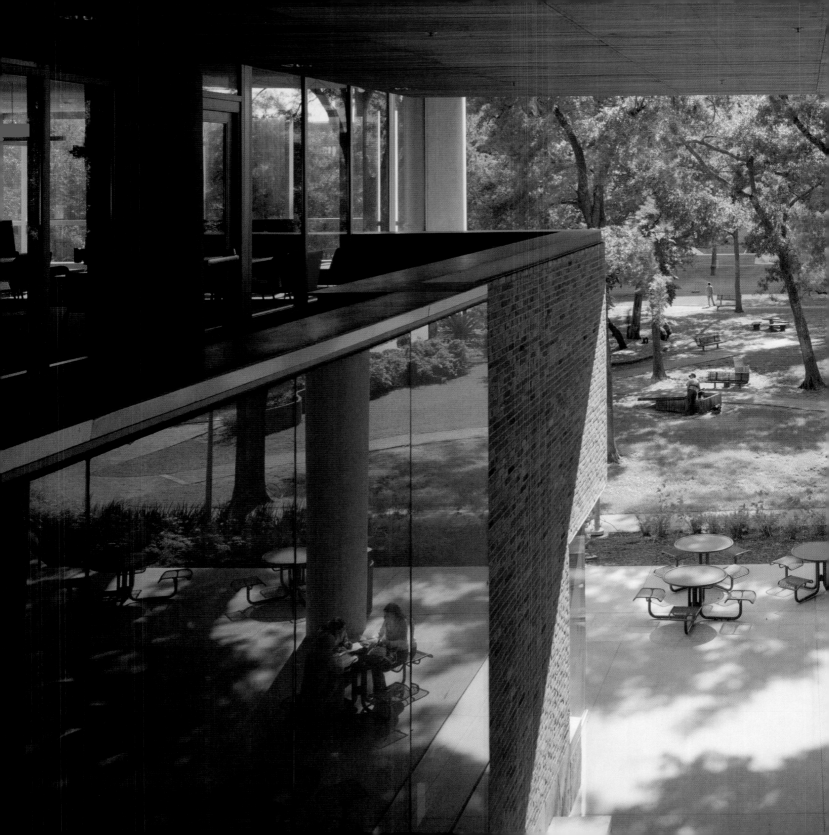

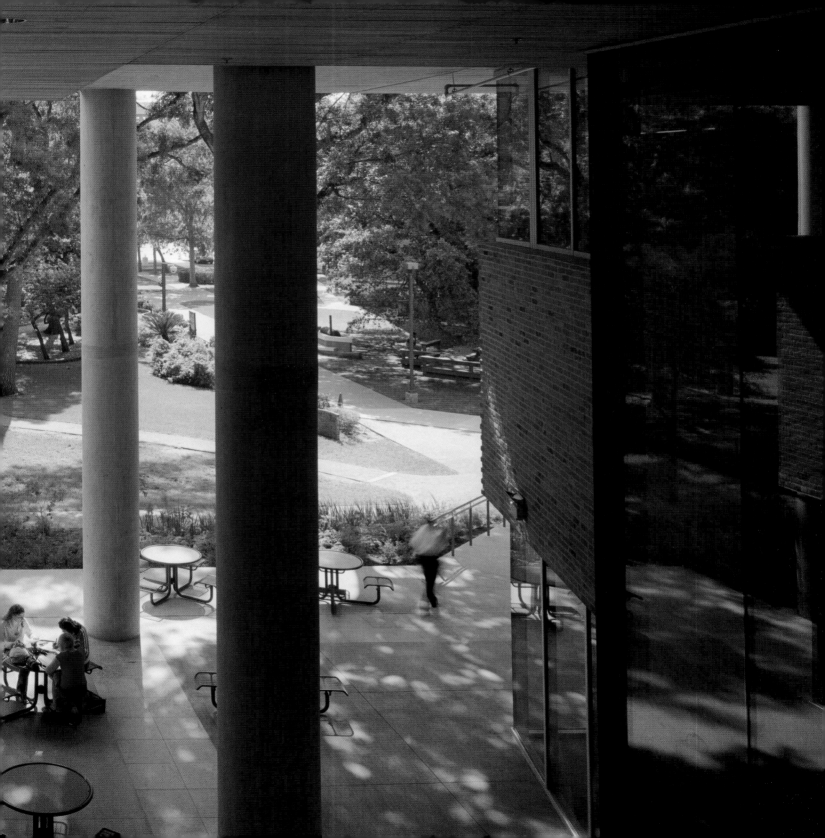

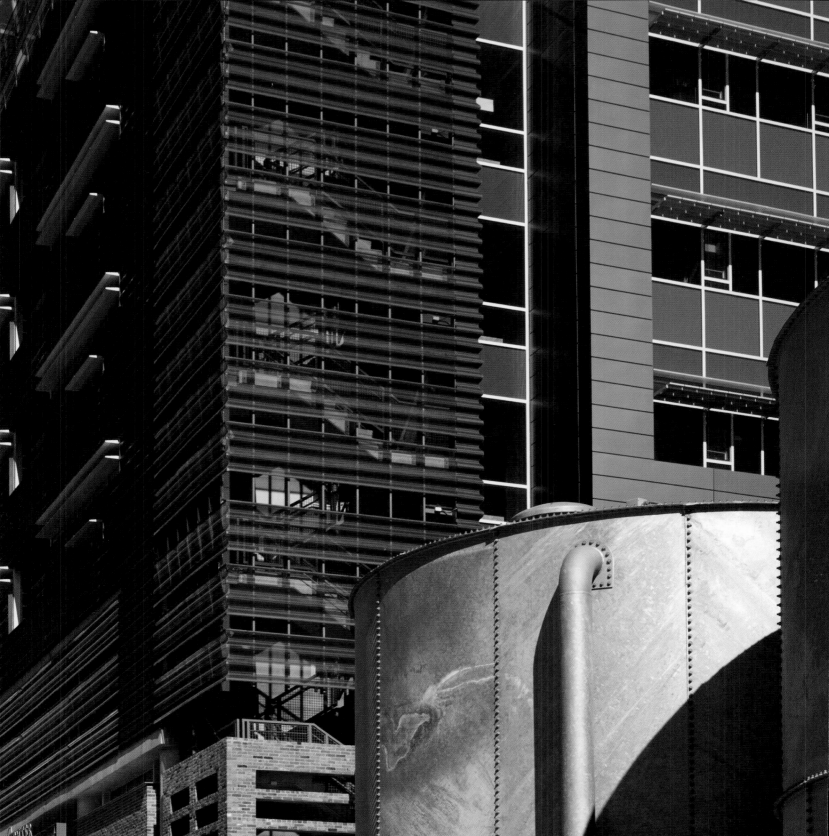

2. WATER EFFICIENCY

Unpredictable weather conditions made protecting water resources a priority. Some seasons bring rain and floodwater, while at other times drought and heat challenge plantings and the landscape. The design approach addresses both of these conditions and reduces the amount of potable water consumed by the building, as well as the amount of wastewater leaving the premises.

The stormwater-management design greatly reduces storm runoff through the use of pervious paving systems, green-roof technology and site design that detains rainwater and slows or delays the discharge rate. Additionally, the facility reduces potable water use by harvesting the non-potable rainwater, or "gray" water, from membrane roof areas for later use. This rainwater is stored in five 30,000-gallon cisterns that capture approximately 826,140 gallons of water annually. This water is used for flushing toilets and landscape irrigation on site and at the adjacent UT School of Public Health. Gray water from sinks and showers is also collected for irrigation and flushing toilets— no potable water is used for either purpose, saving 42,000 gallons of water each month. Waterless urinals and low-flow toilets, lavatories and shower heads further reduce potable water use. The cumulative impact of all of these strategies results in a significant reduction in total water use for the building. Sixty-five percent of the total water used in the facility comes from reclaimed sources. As a result, the building uses 48% less potable water than a comparable, conventional building.

Landscaping and plant materials also play an important role in the water efficiency. Utilizing indigenous, low-maintenance plant materials for the planted areas surrounding the building contributes to a dramatic reduction in potable water use.

To improve flood protection, the first floor is elevated above the 500-year flood line, the building has no basement, and primary and backup power are located on the second level of the service building situated to the south.

LEFT
Ninety-five percent of the potable water demand is met by harvesting rainwater from the roof and collecting it in cisterns for later use.

OVERLEAF
Indigenous plant xeriscaping on the green roof.

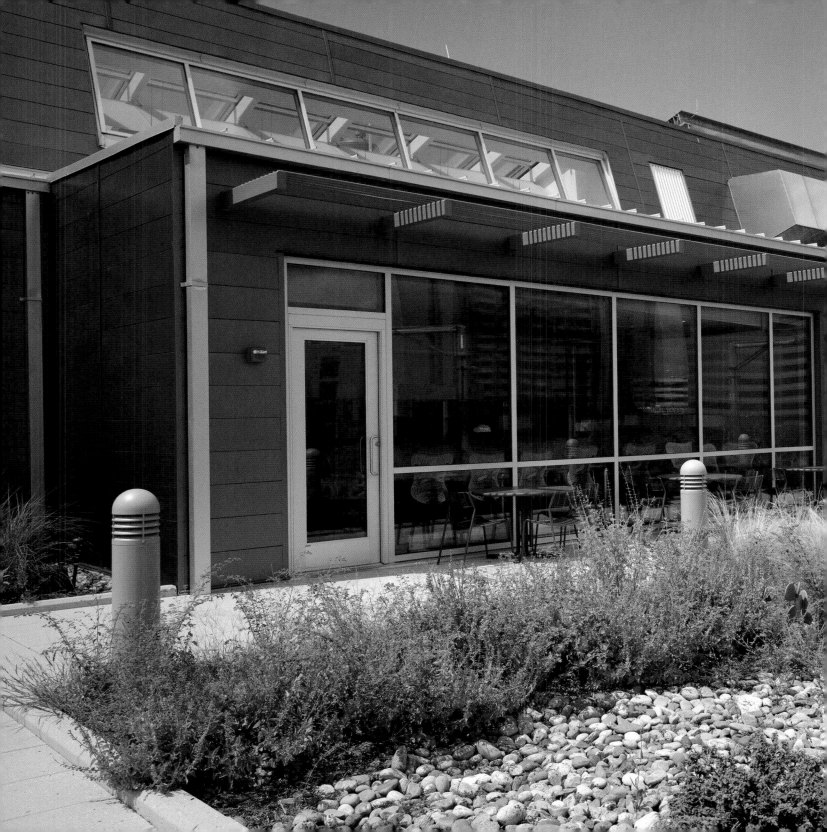

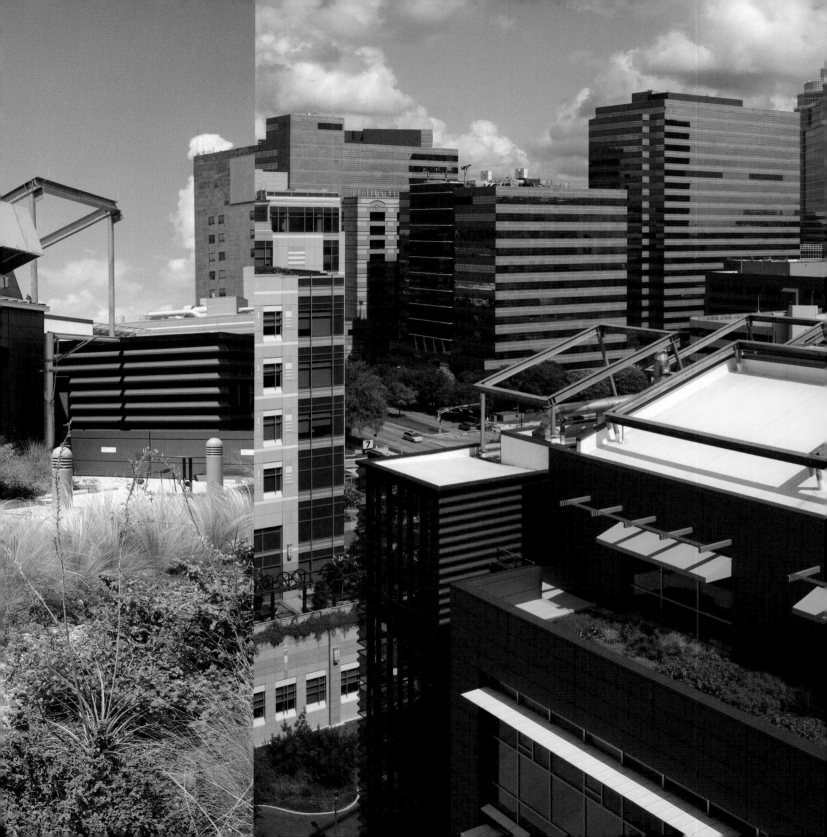

3. INDOOR ENVIRONMENTAL QUALITY

As a facility that teaches healthcare professionals, the building was designed to be a model for how indoor environments can nurture the health and well-being of occupants. Air quality was a consideration for both the occupants of the building and the construction team, who might normally be exposed to volatile organic compounds (VOCs). The team developed an air-quality management plan for the construction and pre-occupancy phases that would benefit the builders and also flush the building of impure air as it was prepared for occupancy. Ambitious goals for indoor air quality were attained through selection of healthy materials, isolating and exhausting the sources of indoor pollution, using a flexible, occupant-controlled ventilation system and adequate commissioning prior to occupancy.

The building promotes indoor air quality and a healthy environment through the selection of materials and access to natural ventilation. The paints, adhesives, sealants, carpets and furniture systems were selected for their low emission of VOCs. A raised floor with underfloor air distribution accommodates workplace reconfiguration as the needs of the program change. This type of air distribution system increases energy efficiency (as air can be delivered at higher temperatures) and provides increased thermal comfort for building users (the air is cleaner and not forced downward), while allowing the building occupants to have some individual control via floor diffusers for increased comfort. The building is both sheltering and nurturing, while retaining an open plan to facilitate collaboration and improve communication between floors, departments and the campus beyond.

All major spaces have access to fresh air through operable windows distributed along the entire façade. The windows provide views and abundant daylight. Meeting rooms and work-spaces on the upper levels open onto three atria with translucent baffles to diffuse daylight. Gathering places (study areas and lounges) look out onto the leafy canopy in the park, and a café is situated along a shaded park space that can be enjoyed whether sitting inside or out.

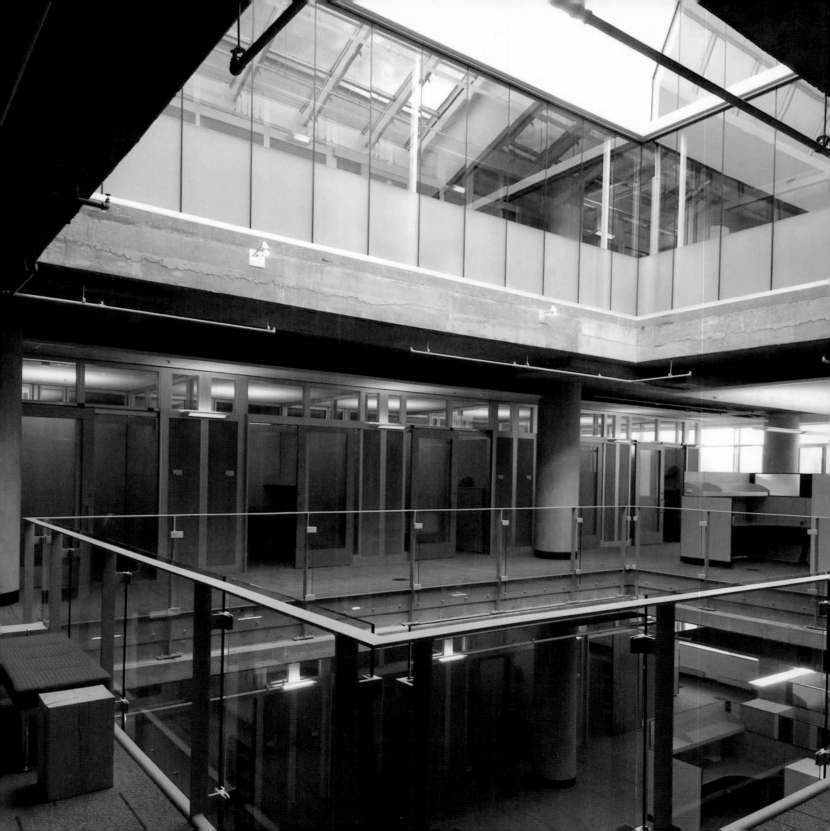

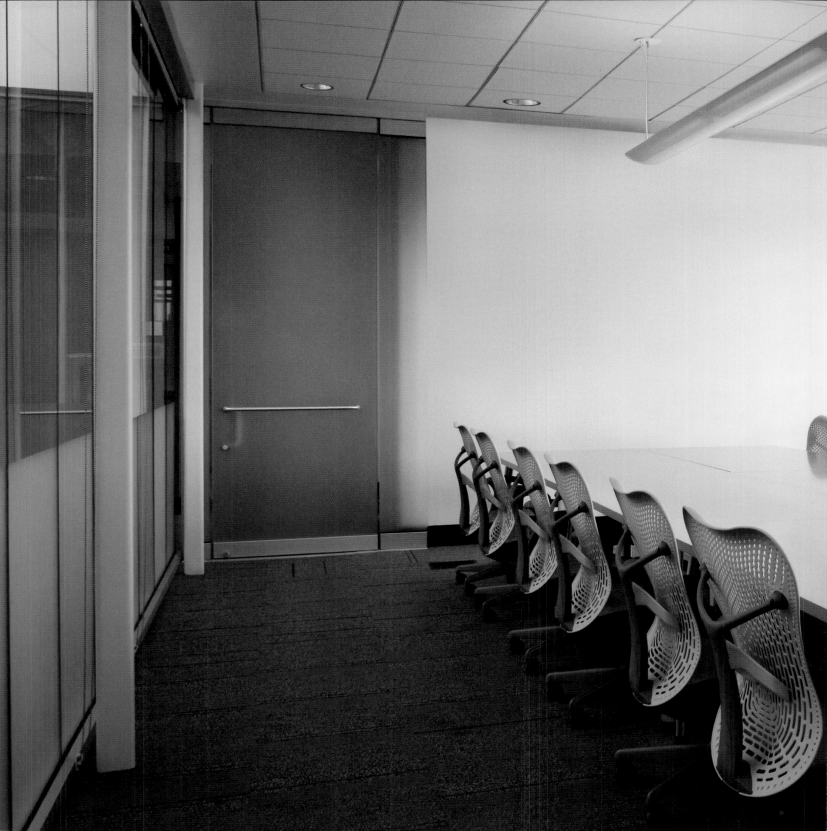

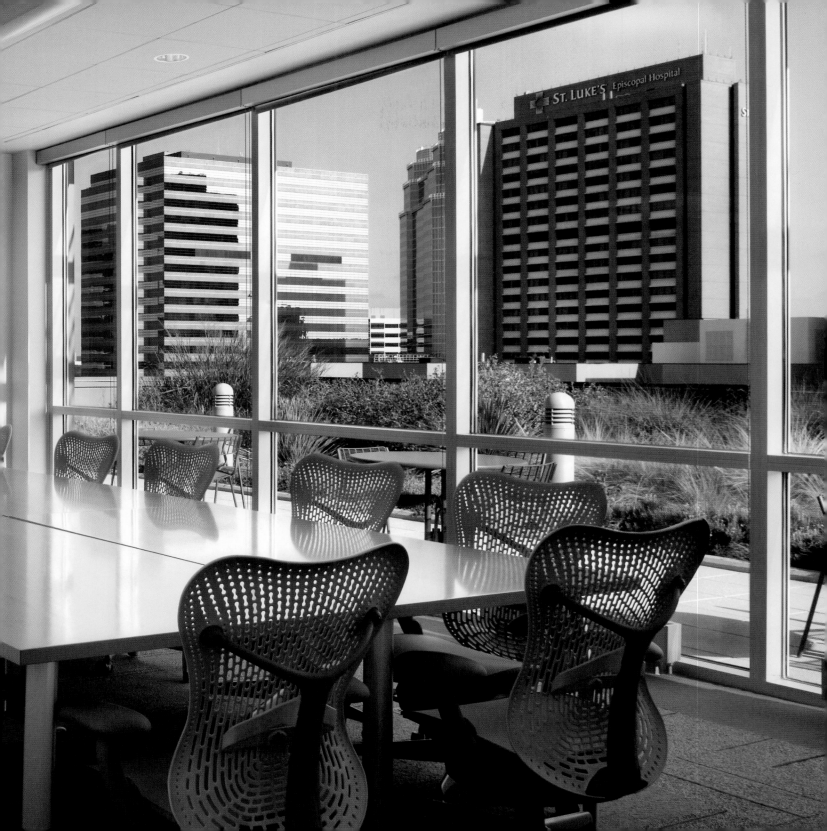

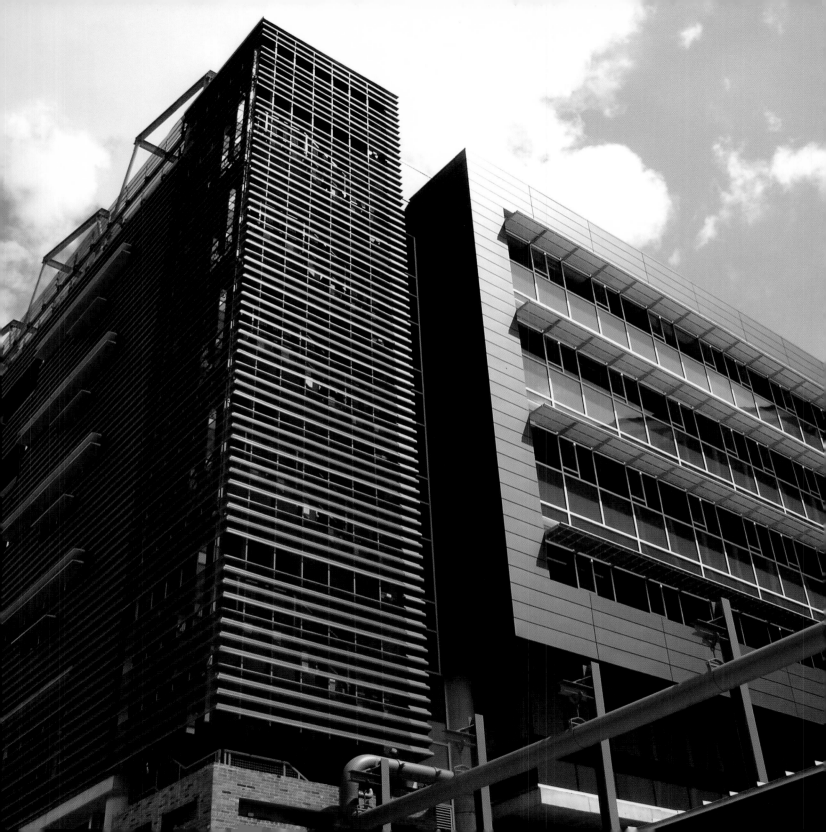

4. ENERGY + ATMOSPHERE

One of the initial goals for the building was to operate at less than 70% of the energy used by the adjacent UT School of Public Health building. A thoughtful envelope design addressed the external factors by integrating numerous passive strategies to minimize direct solar heat gain and maximize use of natural light. The design team's initial studies indicated that the building's primary cooling loads would derive from activities inside the building. People, equipment and electric lighting would generate the primary energy loads. The team also utilized mechanical systems and the lighting strategies to approach these internal issues.

First, the building was designed around a mechanical system that employed a displacement air system using an underfloor air distribution system with low-face velocity coils and chilled water from the central campus system. The benefits of the reduced air-handling-unit fan horsepower and focused cooling of the occupied zone include long-term flexibility, individual user controls, low noise emission and energy efficiency. In addition, this system is "right-sized" according to the energy model data so energy is not wasted to cool the building.

The second important strategy for meeting the energy-use reduction goal was the lighting approach. Daylighting is used throughout the building to provide illumination for as much of the day as possible. This design approach greatly reduces the need for interior cooling to offset the heat generated by even the most efficient electric lighting systems. Occupancy sensors and dimmers are also used to limit lighting loads. The design of the building envelope captures appropriate daylight and rejects unwanted heat and glare with passive strategies including light shelves, vertical fins, window placement and building orientation. Each elevation responds to specific issues related to the sun and, therefore, varies greatly. The glazing percentages on each façade were studied, and performance has been optimized through shading, light-reflecting devices and specific properties based on application (low-e coatings, low

u-value, spectrally selective glass). On the inside, the skylights atop the atria function similarly, allowing daylight, but not heat, to penetrate deep into the building. Beyond these two primary strategies, the building was designed to support the future addition of photovoltaic panels on the roof for renewable energy generation.

Many studies and energy models were used throughout the design process. Both the budget and design energy cases were modeled in VisualDOE (version 2.1E); these models reveal that the integrated strategies worked well in identifying appropriate solutions along the way. The result of these calculations is a $56,142 annual energy savings (43% below the ASHRAE 90.1 design case). The energy cost savings represents the difference in purchased chilled water, electricity and gas costs between the ASHRAE 90.1 case and the building as designed. A fully collaborative process implementing the contributions of many, was extremely important to achieving the design and the final resolution.

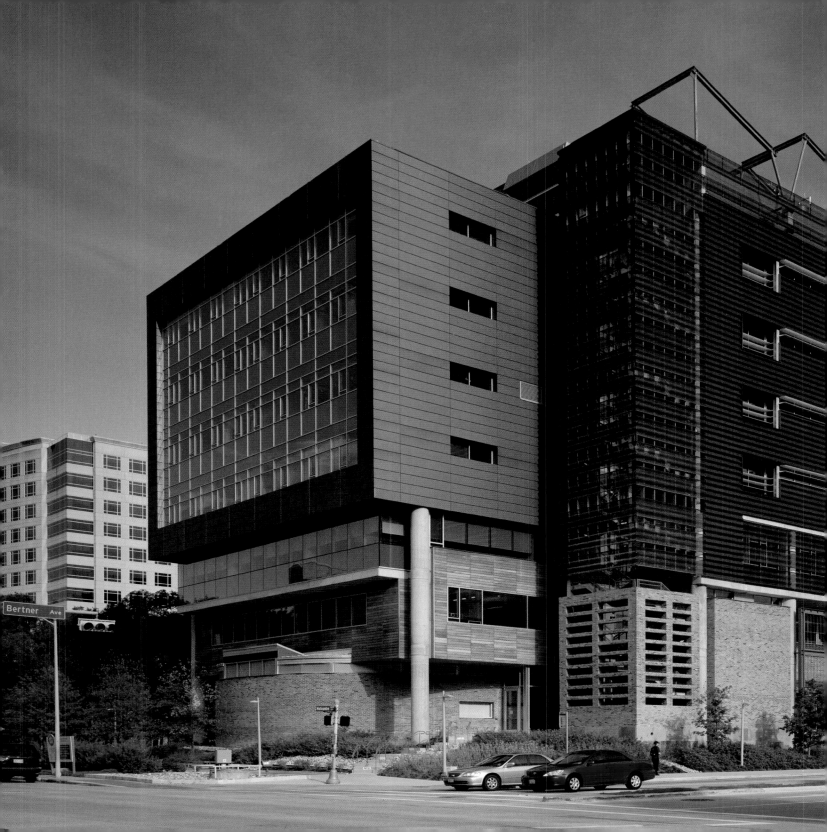

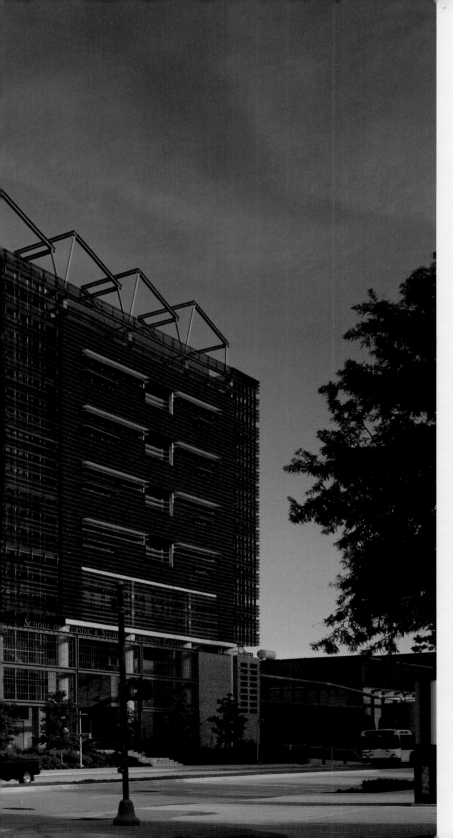

LEFT
The north elevation has approximately
two times the glazing as the west elevation
due to the building's orientation.

5. MATERIALS + RESOURCES

The School of Nursing and Student Community Center has a site-specific South Texas feel indicative of the many local materials used in its design. The design team set out to use locally sourced, durable materials in the highly specialized building skin to encourage long life, promote the local economy and reduce environmental impact. As much as possible, the materials selected have recycled content and contribute to the goal of enduring for 100 years and beyond. Sophisticated life-cycle analysis was done using Baseline Green™, a tool that aids project teams in understanding the upstream and down-stream impact of their decisions regarding materials. The exercise even generated an estimate of how many jobs this project produced or sustained by using local materials. According to the tool, upstream impacts associated with the building were reduced by approximately 2,440 lbs of toxic air pollutants and nearly 300 lbs of toxic water pollutants as compared to the baseline building.

At the time of design, commonly available demountable wall systems did not conform to the standards established for air quality, recycled content, sustainably harvested woods and other sustainable design goals. After research and investigation with the major manufacturers, the design team proposed a process that dramatically improved the sustainability of the wall products. Green specifications were developed that eliminated VOCs, required FSC-certified wood, improved recycled and recyclable systems, reduced waste in manufacturing and made the manufacturing process environmentally better.

The demountable partitions are critical to optimizing flexibility and savings over the life of the building. The manufacturer advised the team regarding finishes and module sizes for the integration of the floor, carpet, furnishings and lighting in an economical way. The team used a 40-inch module as a base, making it efficient to switch door and wall-panel locations. All device locations were pre-drilled and have no panel-to-panel electrical connections allowing pop-in, pop-out interoperability.

The tactile materials used on the lower levels—the local lime-stone base, the brick and the sinker cypress siding—are all reclaimed and come from within a 500-mile radius. The salvaged brick comes from a demolished Austin, Texas warehouse. The cypress siding is cut from sinker cypress logs reclaimed from the bottom of the Mississippi River after sinking over 100 years ago. A high recycled content is specified in new materials such as exterior aluminum panels, window framing, structural steel and concrete. Aluminum siding and window-frame systems are composed of high recycled content, as high as 95%. The concrete structure utilizes fly ash, heavily researched and calculated, to replace 48% of the Portland cement used in traditional concrete mixes and cut carbon-dioxide emissions by roughly 1,800 tons.

The contractor investigated optimal fly-ash percentages for balancing structural performance, embodied energy, construc-tability, schedule impact and cost implications. After a thorough analysis, the results determined that the benefits of utilizing fly ash were significant with no cost or schedule premium. This proved to be a critical process for the project.

Aided by a detailed construction waste-management plan, 75% of the building's total construction waste was recycled or salvaged. The building that once occupied the site was decon-structed, and 4,753 tons of construction waste were salvaged. These materials include concrete, wood, site debris, masonry and scrap metal. A thousand square yards of carpet were returned to DuPont, 14.3 tons of ceiling tile were returned to Armstrong and 50,000 bricks were stockpiled for later use.

RIGHT
Aluminum cladding with recycled content composes the skin and permeable stair enclosure, reclaimed brick, reclaimed sinker cypress siding and concrete structure utilizing 48% fly-ash mixture.

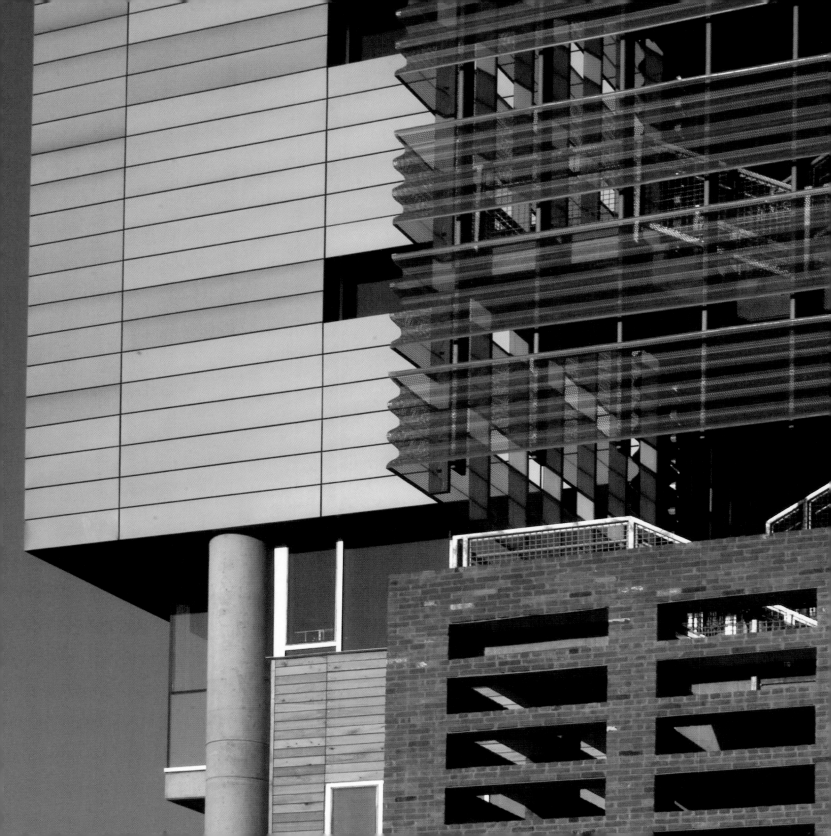

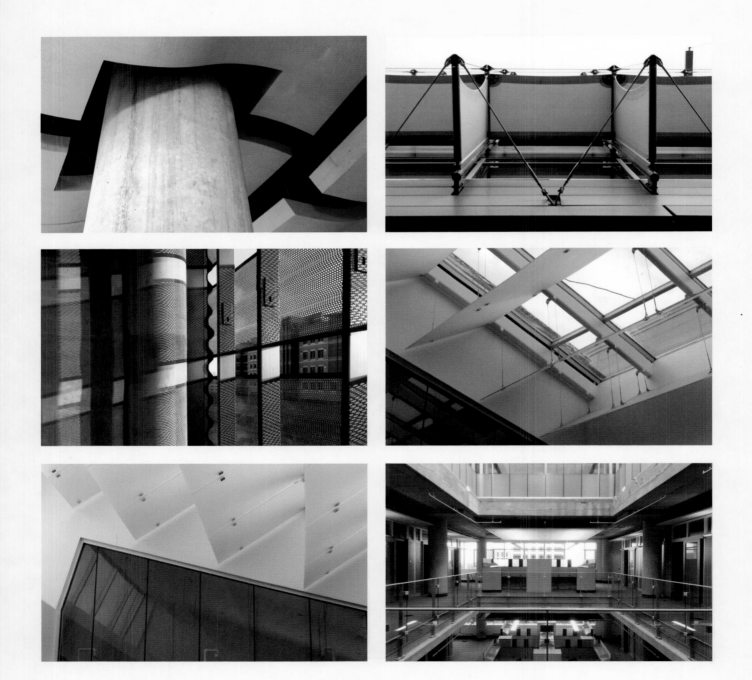

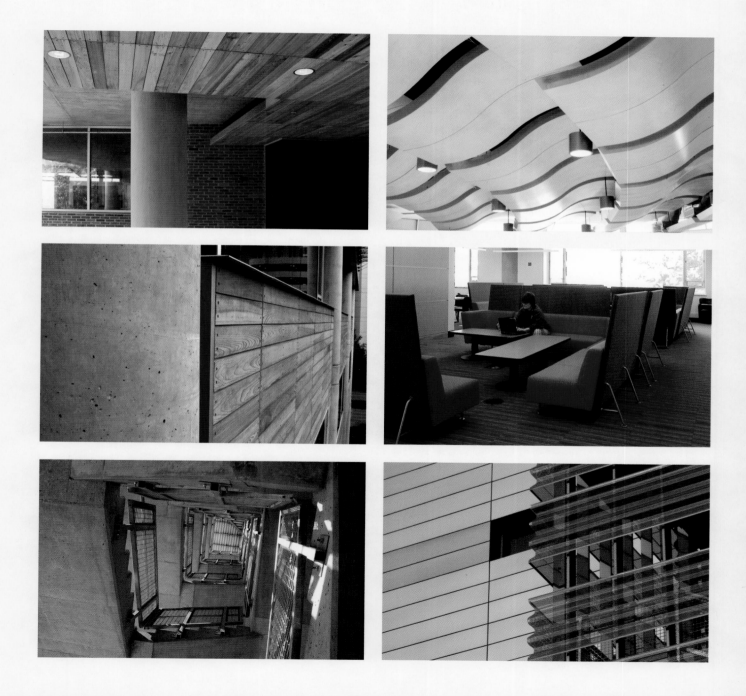

6. INNOVATION + DESIGN PROCESS

The School of Nursing and Student Community Center design team used the U.S. Green Building Council's LEED rating system as a guideline for setting and achieving ambitious goals. The results of this include exceeding the recycled content credits by 25% through the use of recycled materials; exceeding water-use reduction credits by 30%; and mitigating the release of CO_2 into the environment by utilizing a high percentage of fly ash (48%) in the concrete mixture.

From an operational standpoint, the building itself is highly pedagogical, placing on display many of the systems that are integral to its sustainability including rainwater storage tanks, daylighting components and innovative materials. The client's mantra was "you can't sustain it if you don't maintain it," which recognized that design and construction costs are less than 20% of the total cost of ownership. As a result, the building owners conducted a "building systems assessment" that reviewed and assessed design strategies based upon their full cost and several fundamental principles: stewarding resources, doing no harm, benefiting others (present and future) and respecting the environment (with emphasis on CO_2 balancing). In addition, an educational program was put in place to teach about the design of the building.

The results of this philosophy and resulting life-cycle studies support the long-term advantages of flexible, durable systems, including demountable walls, underfloor air distribution, aluminum panel and stone-and-brick cladding, and building-mounted systems for periodic cleaning of the building's exterior. Almost all interior partitions are demountable and designed to be reorganized with ease to accommodate churn or building changes; pre-wired units that utilize "plug and play" technology also mean that cabling changes can be made easily. A raised floor with underfloor air distribution allows individual temperature controls as well as workplace reconfiguration and will accommodate changes to the electrical system over time.

The building was designed for a long life and loose fit. The main structure and its building skin were designed to be highly durable and easy to maintain to ensure that the facility is functional for at least 100 years. In addition to constructing a lasting building that can be easily maintained, the design team moved the exit stairs to the exterior. The exit stairs are naturally ventilated, while shared support facilities reduce the building square footage.

Each aspect of the building, including the exterior envelope, has inextricable relationships with the building systems. For example, the site relates to the interior spaces, and carefully controlled natural daylight impacts cognitive learning and visual acuity, illustrating a few of the building's many interrelationships.

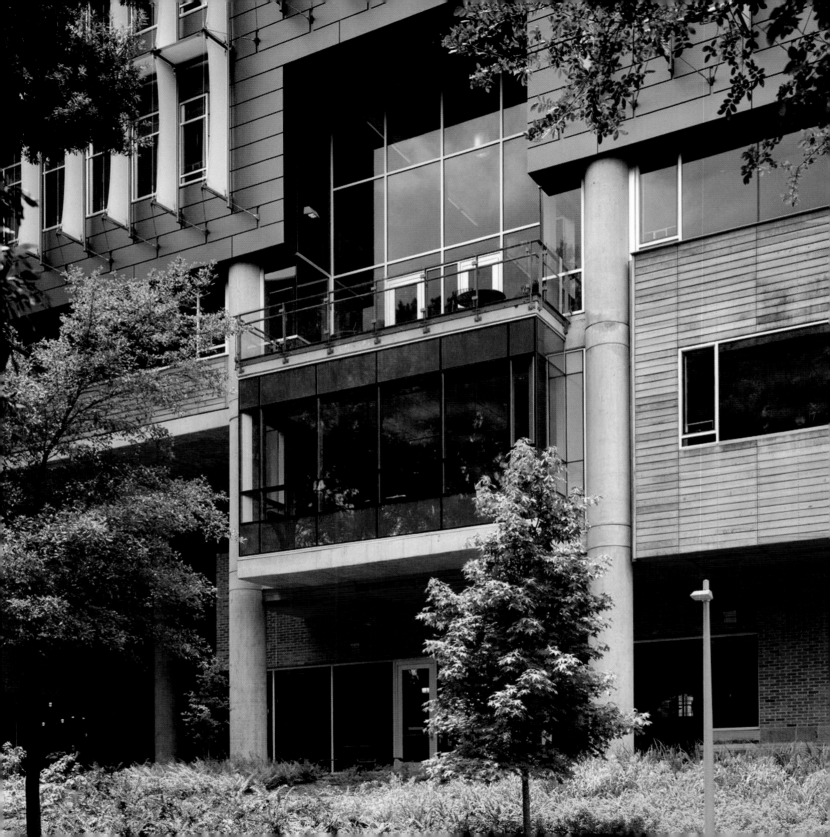

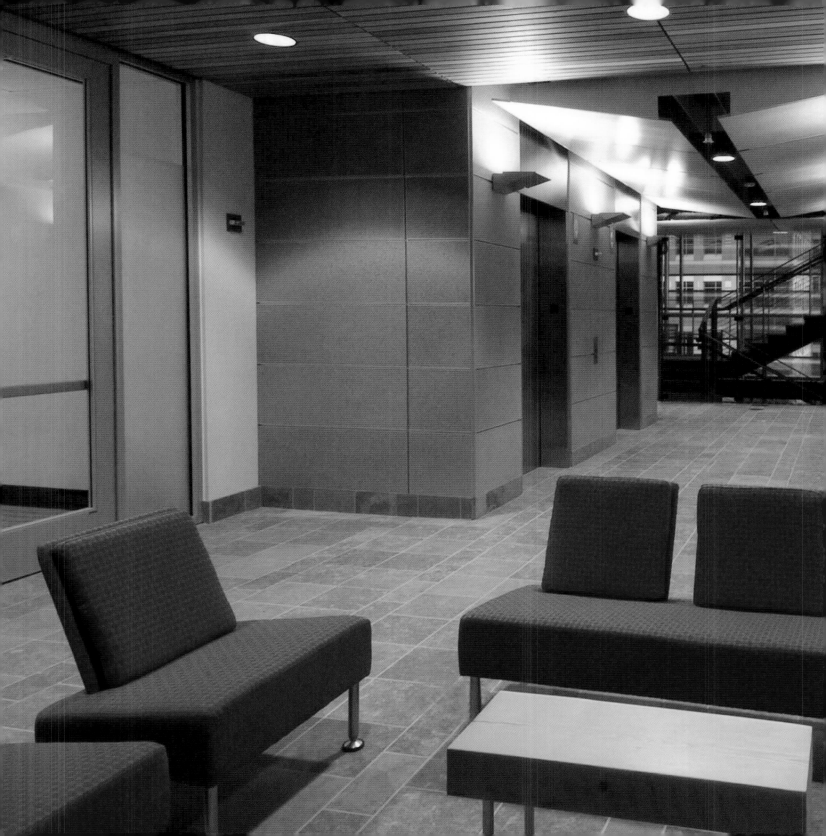

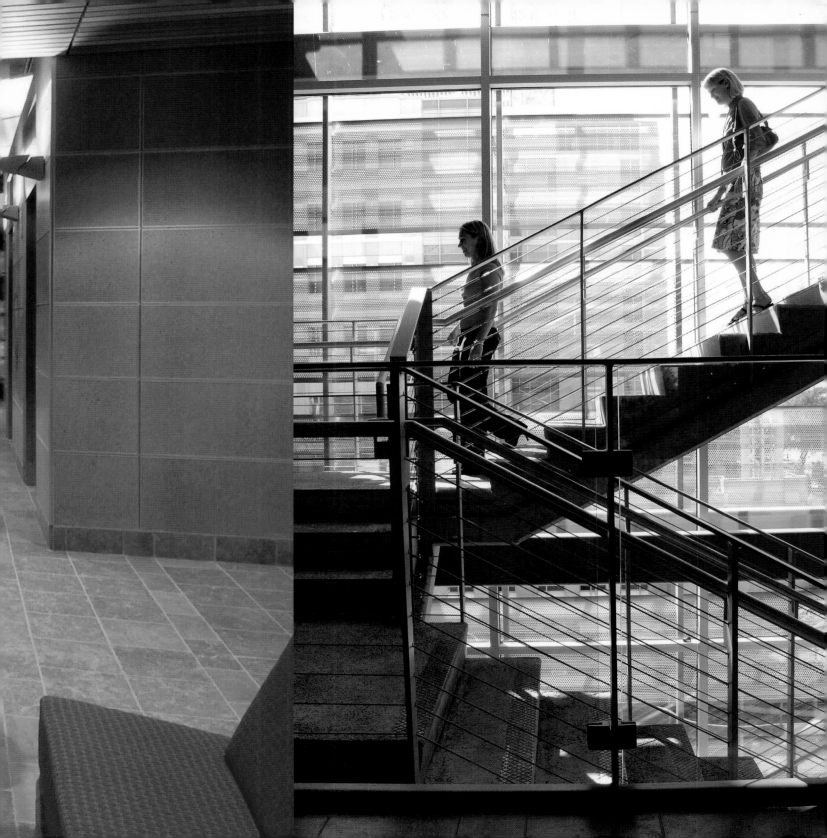

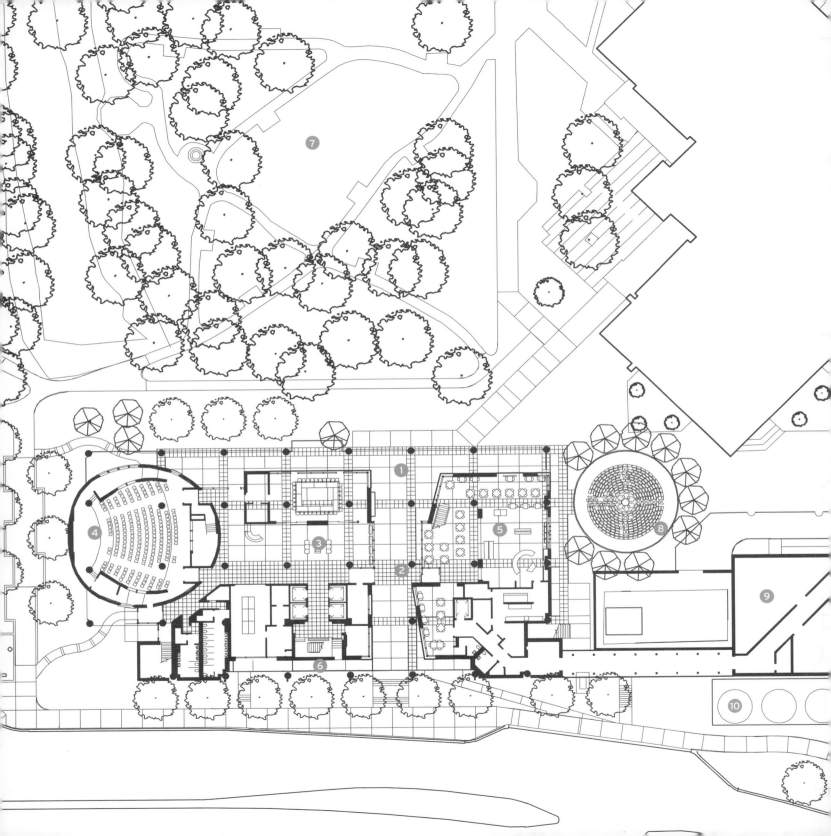

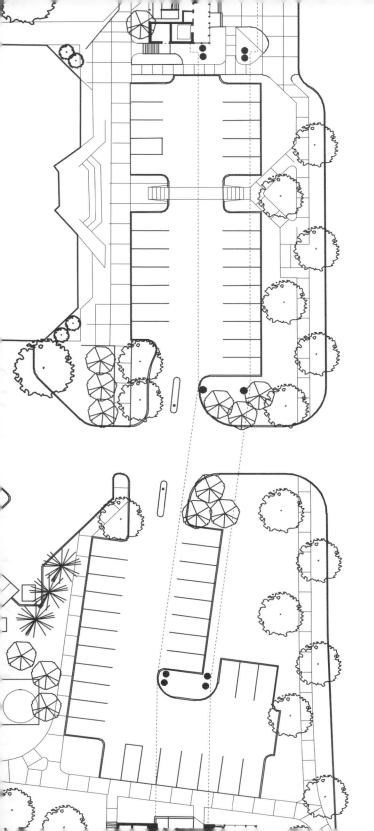

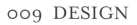

009 DESIGN

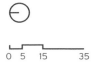

0 5 15   35

1   Breezeway
2   Main Entrance
3   Lobby
4   Auditorium
5   Café
6   Loggia
7   Grant Fay Park
8   Labyrinth
9   Service Building
10 Water Cisterns

0 5 10   20

1   Atrium
2   Offices
3   Lounge / Kitchen
4   Study Lounge
5   Breezeway
6   Bookstore
7   Academic Atrium
8   Classroom
9   Terrace
10 Dean's Office
11 Roof Garden

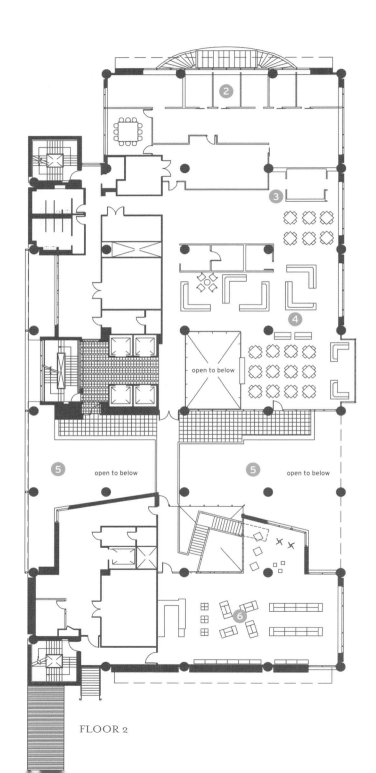

FLOOR 2

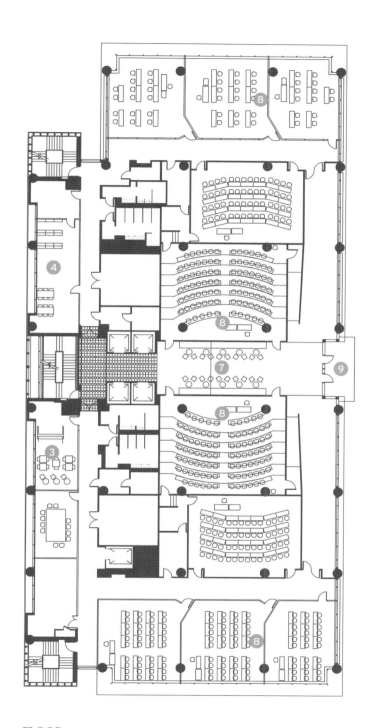

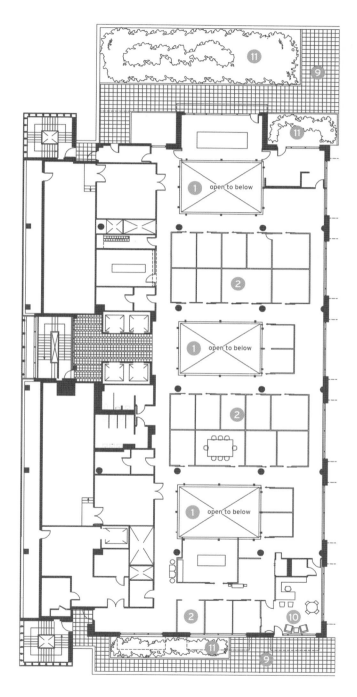

FLOOR 3

FLOOR 8

1   Breezeway
2   Atrium
3   Academic Atrium
4   Offices
5   Café
6   Study Lounge
7   Bookstore
8   Classroom
9   Terrace
10   Dean's Office
11   Roof Garden
12   Auditorium

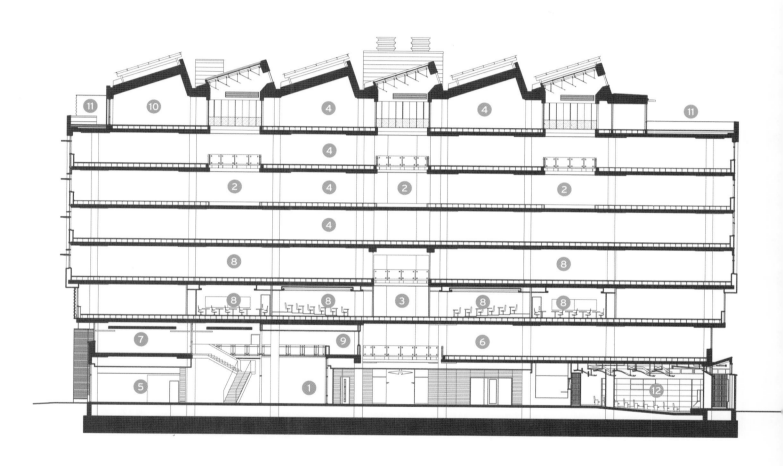

0 5 10   20   LONGITUDINAL SECTION

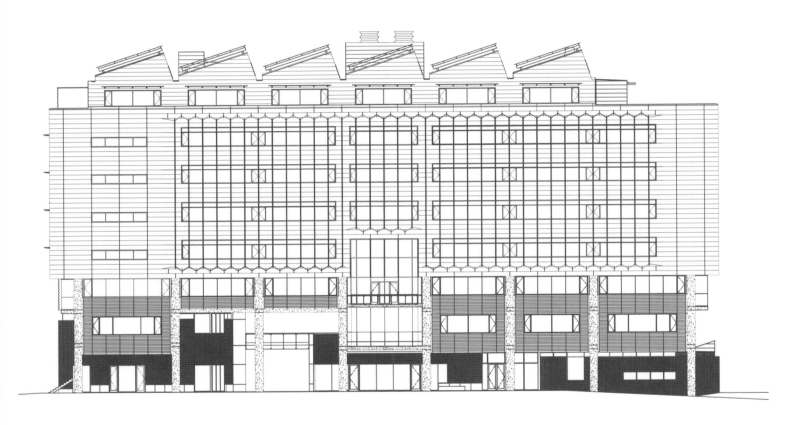

0 5 10   20   EAST ELEVATION

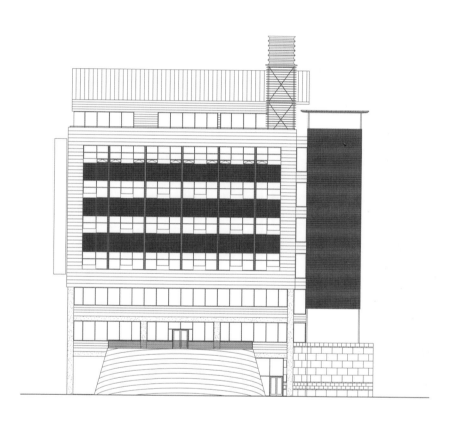

0 5 10   20   NORTH ELEVATION

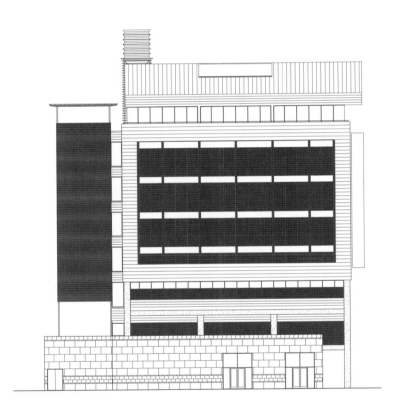

0 5 10   20   SOUTH ELEVATION

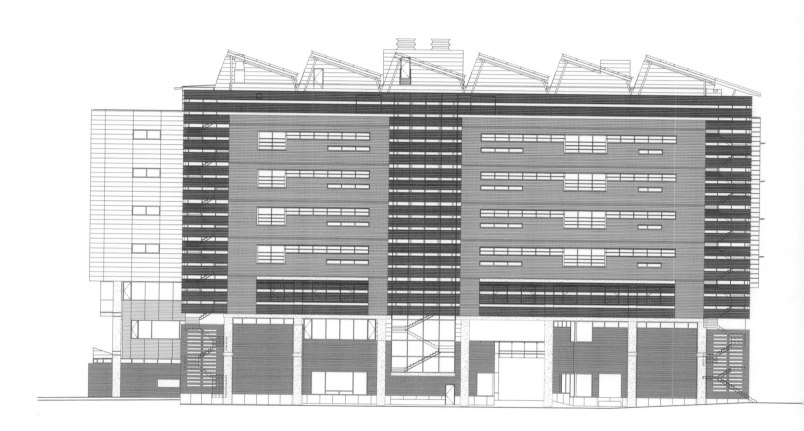

0 5 10   20   WEST ELEVATION

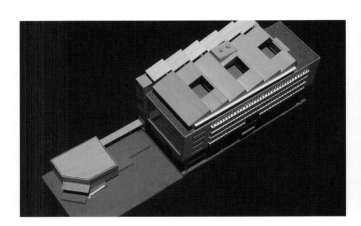

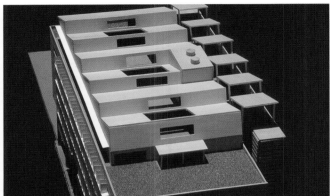

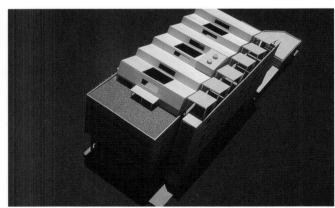

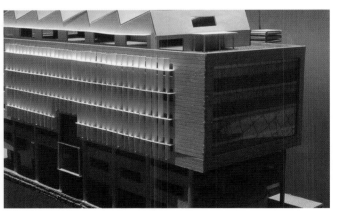

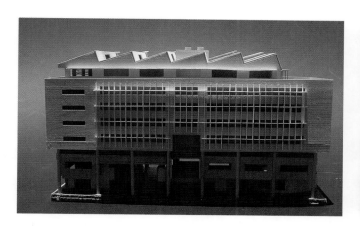
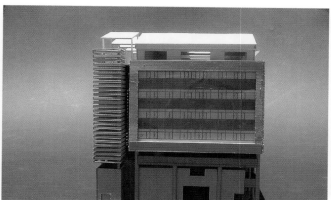
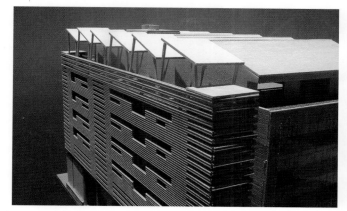
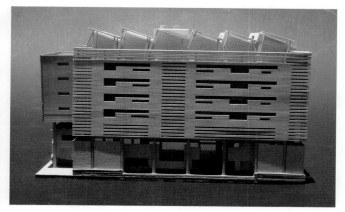

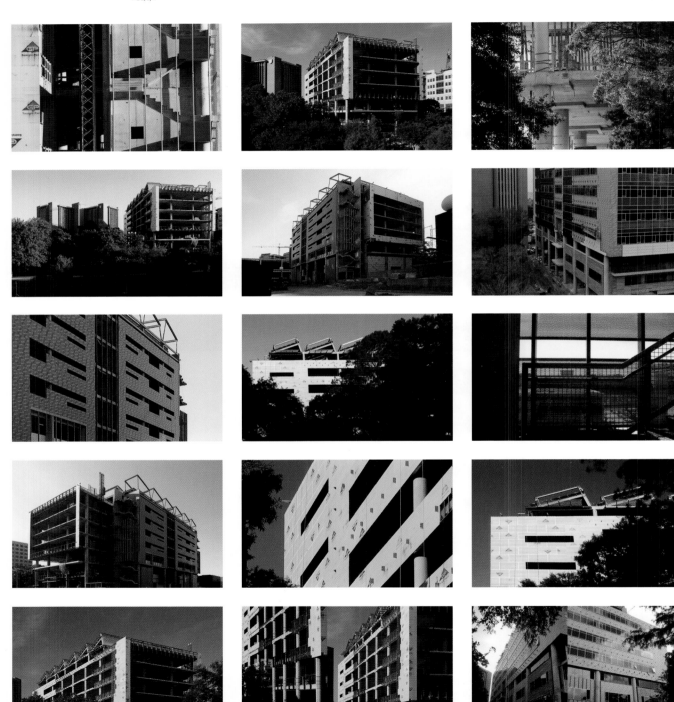

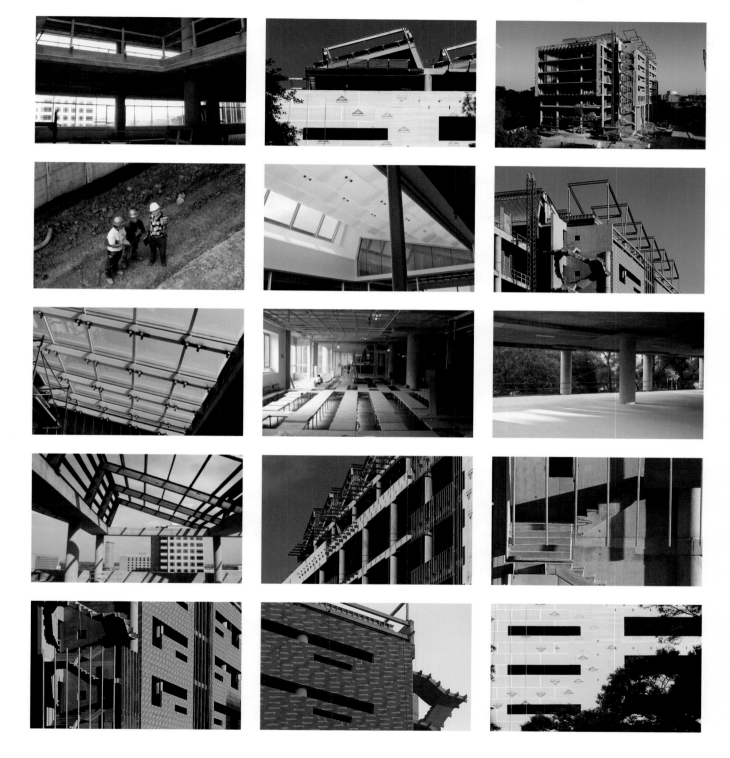

ABOUT BNIM ARCHITECTS :

BNIM Architects is a multidisciplinary architecture and design firm founded in 1970 in Kansas City, Missouri. Throughout its history, the firm has remained committed to its local and regional communities while establishing a national presence as an innovator of design methodologies, sustainability and new technologies in architecture, planning and workplace design.

BNIM's mission is to improve the quality of life for the owner, user and surrounding community through a balance of social, economic and environmental concerns. Without exception, the foundation of BNIM's continued growth and success has been the individuals—client and designer—who share a common vision and who find purpose in helping to create works of extraordinary quality and utility.

Through a process of integrated design, which is both an organized collaboration between disciplines and an interweaving and interconnectivity of building systems, BNIM creates designs that are both environmentally responsible and that achieve the highest level of design excellence. This philosophy, Deep Design/ Deep Green, is embraced by all members of the firm.

As pioneers in the sustainable movement, BNIM and its associates have become known as thought leaders in the industry and beyond. BNIM's passion for sustainability has emerged on the national scene over the past two decades through early involve- ment in the U.S. Green Building Council and other national committees and demonstration projects. Their work helped define the national American Institute of Architects' Committee on the Environment, the USGBC's the USGBC's Leadership in Energy and Environmental Design (LEED®) Green Building Rating System and the Living Building concept.

BNIM's work has evolved to embody the concept of restorative design, which aims to maximize human potential, productivity and health while minimizing the consumption of resources and the production of waste and pollution. They design buildings and spaces that have a benign or healing impact on the site while being environmentally responsible, experientially rewarding and deeply educational for those who interact with them. Their projects demonstrate a belief that buildings and communities are and should be seamlessly integrated with the natural world. This results in structures that respond to and interact with their environment as living systems, celebrating light, water, landscape and natural materials.

Through research and investigation, the use of cutting-edge technology and the execution of solution-driven design, BNIM Architects has gained a reputation for design excellence. BNIM's projects, which include building and workplace design, urban planning and community redevelopment, have won numerous design awards from the AIA and other respected organizations. Included among them are national AIA/COTE Top Ten Green Projects Awards and recognition from the General Services Administration, the American Planning Association, and the International Interior Design Association, to name a few.

bnim.com

ABOUT LAKE | FLATO ARCHITECTS :
Founded in 1984, Lake|Flato crafts architecture that is rooted
to its place. Their buildings are tactile and modern, environmentally responsible yet authentic.

"Lake|Flato's body of work is modern yet not sensational.
Many projects possess that all-too-rare quality of
serenity. It is simple and joyous architecture, rooted
within the regions to which it belongs."

Glenn Murcutt, HFAIA

Lake|Flato's design approach is inspired by the pragmatic
solution of vernacular architecture, the honesty of modernism
and the desire to make each building intrinsically fit the context
and climate while being a natural partner with the environment.
These underlying principles have brought Lake|Flato wide
critical acclaim. The American Institute of Architects awarded
Lake|Flato the prestigious National Firm Award in 2004. In
2006, the firm received two of the Top Ten Green Projects
awarded by the AIA's Committee on the Environment, followed
by another Top Ten Project in 2007. Lake|Flato's work has
received thrity-eight national AIA awards, over thirty Texas
design awards and over sixty local AIA awards. Their work
has been featured in two monographs, over fifty books and is
widely published nationally and internationally. As architects,
educators, environmental stewards and community advocates,
Lake|Flato elevates the public's appreciation of architecture by
creating buildings that seek to protect and restore the natural
ecosystems upon which all life depends.

"In the case of Lake | Flato... their translation into
architecture can serve as a lesson for us all. How a
building stands to the sun, how it welcomes the cooling
breeze—these are lessons in siting. Nothing sensational
or exotic, no visual fireworks of fashion... Timeless
architecture needn't shout; it is more pleasant to listen
to the wind whispering through it."

William Turnbull, FAIA   lakeflato.com

CLIENT TEAM :

The University of Texas System Board of Regents. The University of Texas System - The University of Texas Health Science Center at Houston: Jon Poretto; Rives Taylor; Brian Yeoman; Gerard Marchand; Thomas Roberts; William (Wes) Stewart. **The University of Texas Health Science Center School of Nursing:** Dean Patricia Starck, D.S.N.; Dr. Nancy McNiel; Carolyn Halpin; Maureen Dial; Bob Vogler; Jan Johnson. **The University of Texas System - Office of Facilities Planning and Construction, Houston:** James J. Hicks; Paul R. Zider.

DESIGN TEAM :

BNIM Architects (Architect, Interior Designer): Steve McDowell; Bob Berkebile; Kathy Achelpohl; David Immenschuh; Kimberly Hickson; Ron Ray; Bryan Gross; Darren Oppliger; Christopher Koon; Mary Mermis; Barbara Cugno; Brian Rock; Christina Kohles; Amy Gray; Anil Panchal; Bill Poole; Lacy Brittingham; Eric Morehouse; Mark Kohles; Gretchen Holy; Dirk Henke; Phaedra Svec; Monita Ireland; Sarah Lienke-Nickle; Jay Siebenmorgen; Aralia Sendejas; Gary Jarvis; Maria Morehouse; Jason Lutes; Hande Aydin; Aaron Blumenhein; Christopher Claus; Christi Anders. **Lake|Flato Architects** (Architect): David Lake; Ted Flato; Greg Papay; Kenny Brown; Jay Pigford; Matt Burton; Dale Riser. **Jaster Quintanilla & Associates** (Structural Engineer): Gary Jaster, Scott Francis; Dan Grant; Usnik Tuladhar; Jim Frisch; Steve Hetzel; Jason Andress. **Carter & Burgess, Inc.** (Mechanical & Plumbing): Gary Andrews; Bob Drouillard; Penny Middlerad; Scott Selz; Ron Whatley; Tim Koehn. **Epsilon Engineering, Inc./Edwards and Kelcey** (Civil): Keith E. Smathers; J.Thomas Evans; Gary R. Myers. **Ferguson Consulting** (Electrical Engineer & Security). **ARUP** (Envelope): Alisdair McGregor; Fiona Cousins; Maurya McClintock. **Center for Maximum Potential Buildings** (Sustainable Design): Pliny Fisk III; Rich MacMath; Gail Vittori. **Rocky Mountain Institute** (Sustainable Design): William D. Browning. **Elements, a division of BNIM Architects** (Sustainable Design): Jason McLennan; Monica Rodriguez; Bradley Nies. **Supersymmetry** (Energy Efficiency): Ronald Perkins; Joanne Peden. **Rolf Jensen & Associates, Inc.** (Code): Michael A. Crowley. **Lerch Bates, Inc.** (Vertical Transportation): Jay Popp. **P & W Architects, LLP** (Laboratory): Victor V. Gelsomino; Gerardo Manzanares. **Clanton & Associates** (Lighting): Nancy Clanton; David Nelson; Todd Givler; Dane Sanders. **Coleman & Associates** (Landscape Architecture): Aan Coleman; Thomas Parker. **Worrell Design Group** (Food Service): Rodney A. Worrell; Larry E. Wolfe; Nestor Montoya; Steve L. Wintner; May Boitel. **Pelton Marsh Kinsella** (PMK Consultants) (AV and Acoustics): Howard K. Pelton; Ted N. Carnes. **Walter P. Moore** (Roadway and Parking): Edwin Friedrichs; Charles Penland. **Busby & Associates** (Cost): Kenneth Busby; Claude Eudaric; Bill McCauley; Gwendy Taylor.

AUTHORS :
Steve McDowell and David Lake
Introduction : Andrew Payne and Rodolphe el-Khoury

BOOK DESIGN :
BNIM Architects
Senior Designer : Matthew Alan Stiffler
Project Coordinator : Erin Gehle

PHOTOGRAPHY :
Farshid Assassi, Assassi Productions : 27, 47(TL), 58, 72/73, 93, 96/97 -- Paul Hester, Hester + Hardaway : 14, 16, 20, 23, 32, 36, 40/41, 47 (BL&R), 49, 64, 68/69, 70, 74/75, 76/77, 87, 88/89, 90, 95, 98, 100, 103, 104 (all but BR), 105, 108 -- Richard Payne : Front / Back Cover, 6/7, 8, 42, 44/45, 47 (TR), 55, 62/63, 66/67, 71, 81, 92, 100/101, 104 (BR), 107 -- Filippo Castore : 65, 109 -- Pro Aire Photography : 31, 34/35 -- Mary Watkins : 28/29

FIRST PUBLISHED by :
ORO *editions*
Publishers of Architecture, Art and Design

Gordon Goff and Oscar Riera Ojeda - Publishers
West Coast : PO Box 150338, San Rafael, CA 94915
East Coast : 143 South Second Street, Ste. 208, Philadelphia, PA 19106
oroeditions.com | info@oroeditions.com

Copyright 2008 ORO *editions*

ISBN 978 - 0 - 97938 - 011 - 2

DISTRIBUTION :

In North America	In Europe	In Asia
Distributed Art Publishers, Inc.	Art Books International	Page One Publishing Private Ltd.
155 Sixth Avenue, Second Floor	The Blackfriars Foundry	20 Kaki Bukit View
New York, NY 10013	Unit 200	Kaki Bukit Techpark II, 415967
USA	156 Blackfriars Road	Singapore
	SEI 8EN	
	United Kingdom	

ORO *editions* and BNIM Architects + Lake|Flato saved the following resources by using New Leaf Reincarnation Matte, manufactured with Green-e® certified renewable energy and made with 100% recycled fiber, 50% post-consumer waste and processed chlorine free: 37 fully grown trees, 7,974 gallons of water, 17 million BTUs of energy, 1,744 pounds of solid waste and 2,948 pounds of greenhouse gases. newleafpaper.com

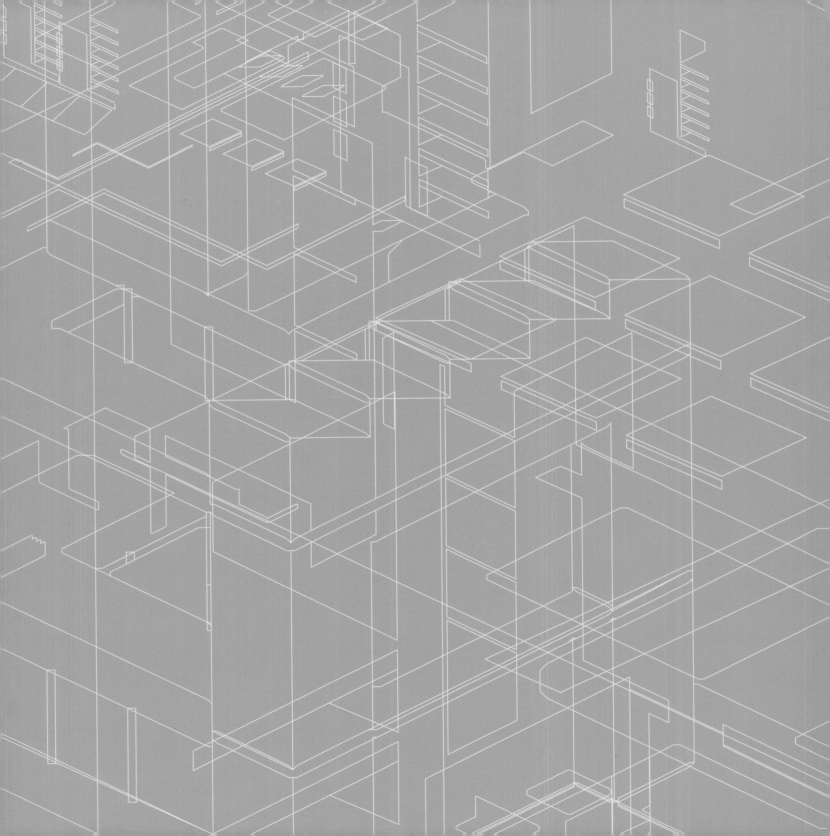